LINDA EVANS
BEAUTY
AND
EXERCISE
BOOK

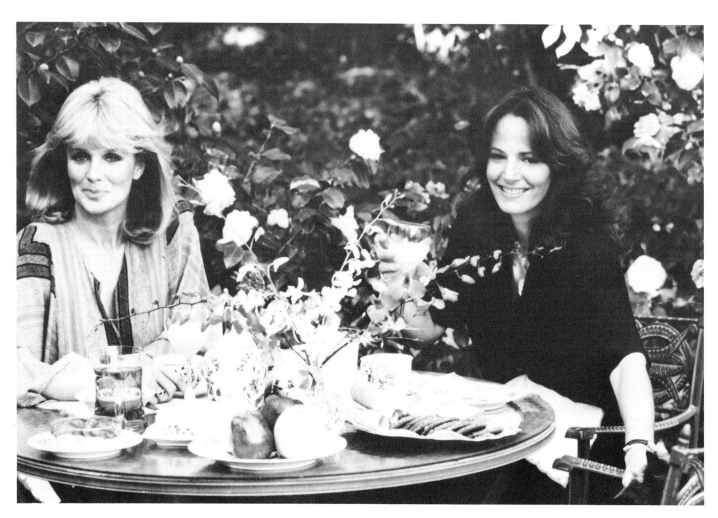

PHOTO BY O. MONSERRAT

LINDA EVANS
BEAUTY
AND
EXERCISE
BOOK

INNER AND OUTER BEAUTY

"I just want to be the best me I can be."

by Linda Evans

COLLABORATING EDITOR: Sean Catherine Derek

ORBIS PUBLISHING · London

My mother and father,
who by their love gave
me the greatest gift of all.
I dedicate this book to
their memory.

ACKNOWLEDGMENTS

I'm eternally grateful to Patricia Sun, for the love and guidance she has contributed to my life and to this project. But most of all for being the brightest light, an example of what we can all be.

To my loving friend, Linda McCallum—thank you for sharing your inner wisdom and knowledge, and for always being there for me.

My dear friend Jackie Eastlund—thank you for sharing your love of God with me, and for helping me through my darkest hours.

Special thanks to Diane Beber for helping me begin my journey inward.

I'm deeply grateful to Reverend Jackie Sorensen, a beautiful woman who knows the truth and helps us to set ourselves free.

To Winnie, my very special friend—thank you for the loving way you inspire us to care about ourselves.

My warmest thanks to Anne Randall, who will always have a special place in my heart. Thank you for being my buddy.

To my brilliant friend, Bridget Hedison—thank you for adding so much joy and wisdom to my life and my book.

To Armando Cosio, an artistic genius—thank you for sharing so much with me.

Thank you Nolan Miller—you've spoiled me forever. Thanks for being my friend and sharing with us.

My very dear Cherie, how can I ever work without you? You're a joy and a pleasure to know. Thank you.

I want to thank Lola, my talented, gifted friend, for generously contributing her knowledge to us.

My thanks to Teressa Reno for graciously allowing me to publish her life's work.

Very, very special thanks to Bunky Young, my oldest friend. Thank you for your encouragement, love, and guidance.

My love and thanks to George Santo Pietro, for keeping his promise, and for sending over the pizzas while we worked on this book.

Thank you Doctor Robert Rosenfeld for taking time out of your busy schedule to help us.

To Shirley Eder—thank you for your inspired chapter.

Thanks to Mia Evans for her time and efforts.

To Mario Caselli—thanks for always making me look beautiful.

Thanks to Bonaventure Inter Continental Hotel and Spa for the use of the photograph on the cover of this book.

But most of all, from the bottom of my heart, thank you Sean— you've made my life and my book better because of your love. I couldn't have written this without you.

Contents

Preface

Initially, when I was asked if I'd be interested in writing a "Beauty Book," along the lines of *The Perfect 40,* I just laughed. I was flattered by the proposal, but the idea of publishing my "Beauty Secrets," was absurd to me.

"Obviously," I admitted later to a friend, "over the last twenty-five years I have learned a great deal about beauty. Or at least, I've learned what works best for me and my friends. I've been taught by the experts, people who have devoted their lives to one particular beauty field.

"Like Lola, who does my facials. She's spent her life studying and practicing her craft. She's literally rejuvenated my skin.

"Winnie is another expert. She knows more about massaging cellulite away safely and effectively than anyone else I've met in the business.

"Over the years, I've worked with so many makeup artists, I've lost count. But Armando Cosio, the gentleman who now makes me up for my endless still-photography sessions, has taught me more about makeup than any of the others. He's brilliant, and his life is beauty.

"Naturally, I've learned a great deal about fashion and clothes from my friend Nolan Miller. After all, look at the incredible designs he does for 'Dynasty,' not to mention his other accomplishments.

"I've worked with many hair dressers in Hollywood and on location, but they have never shared their secrets with me the way Cherie does while we're working together on 'Dynasty.'

"When it comes to keeping in shape, dieting and exercising, there are certain programs I prefer to others. Over twenty years ago I developed a special exercise program that works well for me and makes working out more enjoyable.

"And until I met Reno, my manicurist, my nails were a mess, chipping and breaking. She's taught me the key to keeping my nails strong. But again, Reno's a professional.

"But the truth of the matter is: I believe that beauty is a direct result of our thinking. Naturally, the proper care, exercise, facial techniques, massage, makeup, etc., are very important for all of us. But for me, the secret of beauty is in my thinking.

"Now, if someone would let me detail the marvelous methods I've learned about: letting go of fear, attaining self-worth, learning to be strong without being aggressive, as well as all the other extraordinary ways women can improve their lives, as I have, then I could see writing a book.

"If I could actually share the valuable information I've accumulated from the experts on outer beauty, letting them relay their programs directly to the reader, while incorporating what I've learned about inner beauty from experts like Patricia Sun, Linda McCallum, Reverend Jackie Sorensen, and Jackie Eastlund—and, of course, my personal life experiences—then I'd love to write a book for women."

Well, as you can see, the publishers said, "Go right ahead, Linda."

Introduction

Before we begin, I would like to say to you that I am not a doctor or a psychologist, and I don't profess to be either. I'm simply a woman who has spent the last twenty-five years searching for ways to improve and better myself.

By studying countless different religions and philosophies, and with the help of many wonderful people, in addition to day-by-day life experiences, I've been able to accumulate information that does work to make life more rewarding and enjoyable.

I have divided this book into two parts: *inner* beauty and *outer* beauty, because I believe outer beauty is a direct result of how we feel inside.

It isn't absolutely essential to read *Part One* to be able to apply the outer beauty methods to your life, but it would be far easier to understand how it works for me if you did.

The best way I can think of to explain what I've learned is by sharing my innermost personal feelings and experiences. This is something that I've never done before in magazines or interviews. There was no reason to. But if I can help you to feel better about yourself, I have to share and be open with you.

The one thing that I know for sure, is that *I just want to be the best me I can be.*

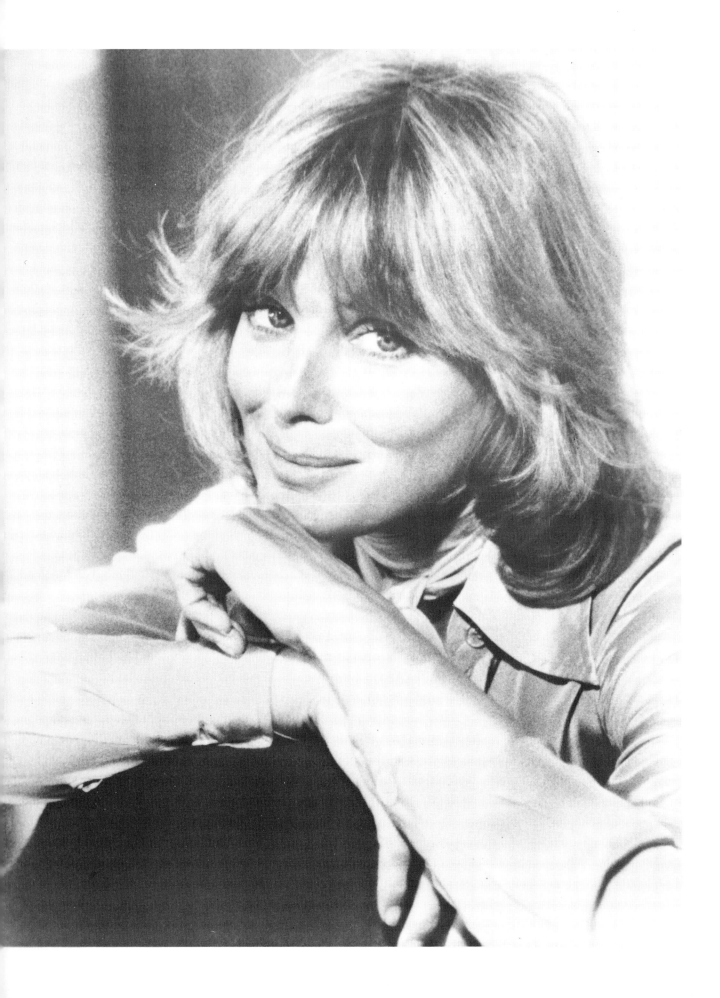

PART ONE
INNER BEAUTY

The Journey Inward

Each of us is a miracle, wonderfully and individually created to be the only one of its kind in the universe.

I feel that life is a gift, an exciting and stimulating adventure. What we do with it, the extent of our happiness, depends on how we choose to look at life. It's really never too late to change our views or adjust our thinking, and it's certainly never too early.

As my awareness expanded, and I learned more about myself, I began to realize that *I am* capable of changing anything I don't like about my life. I believe that all those who want to improve themselves or their lives can do so. But it may take some work.

I've always been told that my attitude in general is extremely positive. I'm simply someone who refuses to become trapped in the negative. I never allow myself to concentrate on the bad; I look for the good in every situation.

I believe that life is a learning experience, both the positive and the negative sides. Each day, we're given the opportunity to grow, to refine our thinking and better ourselves.

Looking for the joy, rather than focusing on the sadness, has helped me in every area of my life. As a result of my thinking, I have a very happy and productive existence.

Even as a child I was positive in the face of hardships. I've always known in my heart that I was entitled to happiness. Never have I believed that I had to suffer, or that life couldn't be a beautiful experience.

Believe me, I'm not saying that I've never been temporarily unhappy, or felt fear, loss, or excruciating emotional pain. Indeed, I have known *all* these sides of life intimately. But I never permit myself to wallow in the negative or the pain.

The journey inward for me was one of the most frightening prospects in the world, because I wasn't confident that I was going to be pleased with what I'd find.

After all, I was already in my mid-thirties and I'd success-fully avoided looking back. Why then should I risk upsetting myself so late? I kept asking myself.

I was torn between wanting to improve myself and wanting to stay where it was safe, where I was comfortable.

In addition to being afraid of what I might find out about myself, I was terrified that if I dug around inside long enough, I might discover something that could turn my entire world around. "Maybe your friends won't love or understand the 'real you': that part of yourself that you seem so afraid to meet." My inner dialogue on this issue was loud and fearfully clear. The process was an incredibly painful struggle for me at first.

Pain is our teacher. Whenever a situation arises that causes anxiety, fear, or pain, I know there's a lesson to be learned. Usually it relates to something I need to understand about myself.

In the past, when it seemed like destiny was leading me down the wrong roads, through painful passages, I'd wonder why I was so far off the track. Then, inevitably, I would find myself exactly where I needed to be to achieve my goals.

Now, when I feel unanticipated pain or confusion, I look for the lesson in the experience, and realize that the pain too shall pass.

Before I could better understand myself and my needs, I had to take the time to investigate who I was, and why. There were certain areas in my life that needed to be changed. For example, I wanted to be a strong woman who was capable of taking control of her life. I knew that I was not exercising any strength or control, but I was unaware of the reasons why. In order to comprehend my patterns, I had to look deep into my past and within myself.

For so many years, people had thought of me in very loving ways. The idea that I might end up altering those loving attitudes was devastating. It could mean that everything that I'd worked for my entire life, to be loved and appreciated, might simply vanish.

Fear

Fear can be a death grip on our persona, especially when our fears keep us from changing. It's so easy to become trapped in old, *familiar* patterns. When we're *used to* the same miserable situations repeating themselves, there's really nothing to fear. In general, we're only afraid of the new.

Facing what I've feared most has been the most satisfying experience for me. I'm the first to admit that I avoided facing fears, for a longer time and with more cowardice than most. However, now I know the extraordinary and rewarding results that confronting the problem can bring, so I'm compelled to stress the value of it.

The longer we avoid dealing with a problem, the greater the fear of it becomes. Our imaginations end up distorting our perspectives and everything seems much worse than it actually is. Regardless of what it is: personal relationship problems, or dilemmas over a need for a change in career, in life-style, or self. When we're afraid of the possible consequences (the unknown results), we're letting fear be the master of our destiny.

If you don't look in the corner, you won't know what's crawling over there, right? And the longer you wait to see what it is, the stronger the fear of it becomes.

Surrendering to our fears is giving fear the power over us. The minute we face the issue, we have some say in it. This immediately removes fear's power over us. It puts us back in control.

I'm only too well versed in fear's dimensions and residual side effects. During one particular incident, fear took me on a journey that taught me a very valuable lesson. Fortunately, the experience ended happily for me. However, it still remains an inexplicable mystery to the respected throat specialist who handled my case. The doctor was left shaking his head in disbelief.

This incident happened last year during the filming of

"Dynasty" (the television series). Each week I receive the script for the following episode, never knowing what my part will entail until I read it. Initially in the show, my character had taken a great deal of emotional abuse without much contest. I have learned many important lessons through the character I play, and this was one of the biggest.

Let me preface this story by saying that when I work I use a method called "sense memory" (similar recall), which means I actually experience the emotional process, the pain or laughter, as I'm "acting," the way many actors do.

That week, I received my script as usual, reviewed it and casually noted to myself that there was one scene that required me to become angry and rebellious (which was new to my character).

The next morning I went to the studio as usual, feeling very good. Everything was going well that day, but as afternoon neared I was beginning to lose my voice. By the time the director asked John [Forsythe] and me to rehearse the "confrontation" scene, I had no voice left at all.

Everyone panicked.

I was immediately sent to one of the most respected throat specialists in town. After a thorough examination, the doctor informed the studio that I would not be able to work for at least a couple of days, but if it was absolutely essential, I could work only half an hour a day. He explained that I had an acute case of strep throat, pharyngitis, and laryngitis. He prescribed medicines and, above all, that I rest and refrain entirely from using my vocal cords.

That night when I got home, I meditated. After my meditation I began thinking about the day's events. It quickly became clear to me that I had avoided confrontation all my life, at any cost. I realized that I desperately needed to learn how to stand up for myself. As hard as I tried to avoid that experience in my life, I was suddenly forced to face it at work.

The next day I went to the set and prepared to work. I told John and the director that I was ready. I did the scene. My voice was there for me, I was completely well.

Later, I called the doctor and told him that I was fine and had worked all day. My "illness" was very real. The cause was also very real to me. However, the cure was letting go of my fear. Whispering for a week or an evening couldn't have made any difference. Until I was able to handle the meaning behind the words, my fear kept its hold on my throat.

My cowardly indecision, to journey inward or stay safe, was a very difficult period in my life. My more intuitive friends all agreed that I was avoiding a valuable source of information. They said that looking inside, looking back and seeing the roots of my fears, could help me learn the truth about myself.

Finally I had to gather my courage and lean on my faith, because I knew in my heart that there were too many unanswered questions and too many situations that were repeating themselves. I needed to know why.

Generally speaking, my life was very nice, but I wanted to improve myself; I wanted to know why I was so reluctant to take complete charge of my own destiny, and reluctant to be strong and in control. And, of course, why had I been divorced twice already?

What was my program for failure? I kept asking myself. I'd made countless excuses for not delving into my past before, primarily insisting that "I'm extremely happy, for the most part." Which was true. "There just can't be anything from my childhood affecting my present-day life."

At first it even appeared as though I had successfully and permanently blocked out all the painful events in my childhood. Actually, I had filed them away so deeply in the recesses of my mind, never paying conscious attention to them again, that I practically had to pry them out.

Overcoming Childhood Programming

We should all look to where the old is interfering with the new. Remembering that in order to heal the scars and erase the "old tapes" (conditioning from past experiences), we must go after the problem knowing we can overcome it. Do *not* fear failure, or you may indeed fail. Experiences in our past do influence our present, whether we consciously acknowledge them or not.

I happen to believe that we choose our parents for the lessons we need to learn. However, whether you believe that theory or find it absolutely absurd doesn't really matter. But if you blame your childhood or your parents for the negative state of your life today, then it's probably time to look back and begin changing your thinking.

We can't blame anyone else in life for our failures and disappointments. Neither Mom nor Dad, sister or brother, spouse or friend. We must go inside ourselves for the answers, and take responsibility for our own actions. I don't mean condemning ourselves for our mistakes, but investigating instead who we *were*, who we *are*, and most of all *who we want to be.*

Believe me, it's never too late to change our thinking. I've made incredible changes at different points in my life.

Sometimes changing a thought pattern can be delightfully simple. It all depends on how much fear is entailed, and how many times the painful pattern repeats itself, and, of course, how much the results will mean to you.

An alteration in my thinking was essential; after all, I was the girl who was going to be happily married till death us do part, spending my life with one ideal man, raising a wonderful family in a picture-perfect home. Or so I thought.

How then could I have failed at two marriages? I decided to find out, no matter how difficult or painful it might be. I had to stare the issue in the face; only then could I change my thinking and alter the patterns.

I grew up in a very modest little house in North Hollywood, California, with my mother, father, and two sisters. We didn't have much money, but I was a very happy child. I've been able to discern that being poor never bothered me consciously or subconsciously.

My main purpose as a child and later as an adult was to be loved. I avoided confrontation no matter what I had to sacrifice. To me, the idea of being direct and assertive meant I might be inviting a negative response, perceived as a form of rejection. What was so frightening about rejection to me, especially as a child, was that I unconsciously linked it to my value as a human being.

I believe that most women, at least to some degree, know what it's like to block their own power (to keep from verbalizing their truth) to achieve or maintain peace. (This is a subject I will elaborate on a little later.)

I'll never be sure exactly when my pattern actually began, but I do vaguely recall an incident when I was very young, which may have launched it.

One afternoon, coming home on the school bus, I managed to get into a minor argument. When we reached my house the driver told my mother that I had misbehaved.

That night, everyone in the family, from my grandparents right down to my older sister, made an enormous production over my behavior.

Apparently, little Linda was expected to be sweet, loving, and, above all, *passive and submissive.*

Whatever actually happened to me really isn't the issue. What's essential is to recognize the repetitious pattern so the problem can be rectified. Whether you're able to pinpoint the source of the programming is almost irrelevant. We should always look to see what's there, but recognizing the actual pattern is the key.

So very early on, I'd resigned myself to being passive and submissive at any cost. Then when I was fifteen, my mother gently broke the news to me that my father was dying of cancer.

At that age I was utterly unable to cope realistically with the situation. What I did instead was virtually ignore, block out, the fact that my father was really going to die.

Every day, before and after school, I'd go into my father's room to see him, never allowing myself to think, even for a minute, that Daddy was really going to die. I just pretended that he had to stay in bed for a while, but that eventually he'd be fine.

Naturally, when my father died, my innermost feelings started attacking me: Had I been there for him? Did he know how much I loved him? What should I have said to him that I couldn't say now?

A major part of me felt that I'd abandoned my father, while another part of me felt as though I'd been abandoned.

Whatever lessons I should have learned from my father's death were ignored. The pain and guilt were too much for me to deal with, so I immediately buried the entire experience. I *never* permitted myself to think about it again. I literally locked it away, blocked it out for twenty years.

Until I was thirty-five, I didn't know, I wasn't even cognizant that I was blaming myself for abandoning my father. For the most part, I was unconsciously determined that I'd never abandon anyone I loved again. No matter what!

Forgiveness

Once I'd faced the issue and recognized the problem I was having with abandonment in connection with my father, the next step was forgiveness. I had looked into my past and had seen what was at the root of my patterns. Then I had to forgive myself totally and completely, accepting that at fifteen I had been doing the very best that I was capable of doing.

There's never been a time in my life that I didn't want to do the very best I could at that moment. We're all doing the best we can under the circumstances.

No matter what we've done in the past, as children and young adults, we must accept that that was then, and it's over and done. We can't change the past. Who we are today and who we want to be tomorrow are things we *do* have control over.

Forgive yourself for the past so that you can love yourself now and tomorrow.

Without my knowing at the time, the unconscious guilt pertaining to my father's death had its effects on both my marriages. The combination of old guilt and the fear of being strong was dictating my destiny.

Many doctors say that when one or both of your parents die, you're forced to face reality more readily because your "safe base" is gone.

I was twenty-nine when my mother died, and the loss absolutely devastated me. But again, instead of searching my soul and coping with what her death really meant to me, I forced myself to block it out completely. Without my mother and father in my life, I just leaned harder on the man in my life (my first husband), and I further encouraged him to decide everything for me.

Obviously, some men thrive on taking control. But sooner or later, fate pushes us into growing up and taking hold of our happiness. Believe me, I know from experience!

My first marriage ended abruptly. We had been together for nearly ten years when one day my husband fell in love with a seventeen-year-old girl and the marriage was over. Quite suddenly I was forced to be alone; I had no alternative.

For the first time in my life, I had to take charge of my own destiny, make my own decisions, like it or not. This undertaking would have been considerably easier had I begun during a calm period in my life rather than amid the chaos of divorce. Nonetheless, the feelings of abandonment and failure, compounded by the precarious position of my self-worth, coerced me into some serious self-analysis.

Fortunately, my faith in God and my basically positive nature enabled me to go forward, instead of becoming trapped in a somewhat warranted depression.

Learning How to Use My Inner Strength

The first seeds had been planted toward the growth of my strength. Giving up my first husband was a major turning point in my life.

At thirty-one, I could no longer escape taking care of myself. But it wasn't until my second divorce that I truly acknowledged my problem. My second marriage ended after three years, primarily because our dreams were not the same; we simply had different goals in life.

One thing was certain: I needed to do some serious soul-searching to find my strength. The concept of being strong and recognizing my inner power has swept through every part of my life like a tidal wave, changing my perspective of everything. I can't overemphasize the value this lesson has had in my life. I know if I hadn't taken the time to discover my strength, I would not have been able to cope with my success today.

So many women believe that in order to be feminine they must be submissive. I was finally able to ovecome that misconception with the help of two very dynamic women: *Linda McCallum* and *Patricia Sun*.

I've been extremely fortunate through the years to have been befriended by several spiritual, knowledgeable, and gifted professionals: people whose life's work is helping others to help themselves. Many of you, I'm sure, are already familiar with some of their work via television, radio, and personal appearances. However, for those of you as yet unfamiliar with Linda McCallum and Patricia Sun, I'm privileged to introduce them to you now.

Although they're both in the process of completing their own separate and individual books, I'm very grateful because they've graciously consented to allow me to share some of the valuable information that helped me grow.

About seven years ago, a friend of mine urged me to make an appointment with astrologer Linda McCallum. My friend

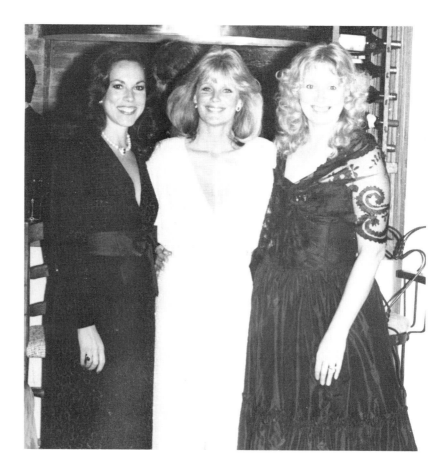

Linda McCallum (left), Patricia Sun, and I at my house, New Year's Eve 1982.

explained that in addition to being an excellent astrologer, Linda was also highly intuitive, which made her readings very special.

After the lovely buildup, I was very excited about the reading. But when it began, I wasn't sure if I wanted to stay or run for the door. What Linda said struck a raw emotional nerve.

"You're a woman who's blocking her own power because you're afraid of it," she said calmly. "You associate being strong with being masculine. This frightens you. But you are very strong, whether you admit it or not."

Throughout the entire reading I argued with her, insisting that she had made some kind of error in my chart.

She smiled patiently and continued. "Most of the pain in your life is a result of your giving your power away to other people. You simply refuse to be strong or assertive. Rather than taking control of your own happiness, you give the responsibility to someone else.

"Whether it be a man, a friend, or a situation you refuse to be the one who makes the decisions. Thus, you won't be the one who makes the mistakes. You sacrifice your happiness to avoid being who you really are: a strong, powerful, and very capable woman."

An hour-and-a-half later, I left feeling confused and disturbed, sensing there was truth in what she'd said and aware of my resistance to it. Linda McCallum had zeroed in on an issue I had avoided all my life.

During the reading Linda expressed her insight regarding my first marriage (which had already been dissolved) with incredible perception, and with no help from me.

I was unable to block out what she'd said, because I knew she was right; I had given my power away at every opportunity. Eighty percent of the time I was very happy doing it. Actually, I was quite good at being the passive, submissive, loving woman I was expected to be. And I was usually comfortable in that place.

It was obvious that the time had come to learn how to become strong without being harsh or aggressive. I phoned Linda McCallum, apologized, and admitted that she'd been absolutely accurate about everything she'd said.

"Now what am I supposed to do?" I asked. It had taken every ounce of courage I had just to admit I wasn't weak.

Linda put me on the course that eventually led me to Patricia Sun.

Again through the strong recommendation of a friend, I found myself sitting in front of a woman who would help me overcome my phobia of taking control.

Patricia is so spiritually evolved and intuitive that it's truly awesome. She's probably the strongest woman I've ever met, and yet she's delicately feminine. She is a teacher and a healer. We met during one of her weekend seminar/workshops and have been dear friends ever since.

One of the most important things I've learned with Linda and Patricia's help, coupled with personal experiences, is that you can handle any ordeal that comes along, just as long as you don't compound the problem by making it someone else's fault. Wasting your valuable energy finding someone else to accuse does nothing to solve the problem. This is part of the process of reaching your full potential and your inner strength.

Judgment

Beauty is eternity gazing at
  itself in a mirror.
But you are eternity and you
  are the mirror.
  —*The Prophet,* Kahlil Gibran

"Everyone you meet is your mirror." This ancient Chinese saying was first introduced to me by Patricia Sun. Since then I have applied the meaning behind these words to my everyday life. The "mirror" has helped me enormously to grow.

Patricia originally suggested the mirror concept after I'd mentioned how, from time to time, I'd encountered a personality that really brought out a negative response from me. I explained that I didn't like wasting my time feeling uncomfortable about someone else's behavior. She explained that if I used the "mirror," I could turn the same experiences "from emotionally judgmental dead ends into empowering learning processes. An unpleasant encounter can become a positive realization." She added, "Blaming someone else solves nothing, and leaves you feeling powerless. Observe and you become wise, compassionate, and empowered through your awareness." She was absolutely right.

The concept of the mirror is very simple: When we have a strong reaction to people, both friends and strangers, it's quite often a mirror, or a reflection of what we like and dislike about ourselves.

When we encounter someone whose behavior disturbs us, many times it's because this individual reflects an unresolved problem of our own: something that we may consider a personal fault, or something that we don't understand or wish we were better able to deal with.

Naturally, the mirror can also work in reverse: You may meet someone you really like who is reflecting your assets, or characteristics that you're proud of.

I strongly suggest that you exercise this concept in your daily life and see if you don't notice yourself in the mirror . . . You may find, as I did, that you don't become nearly as angry at your own reflection. And that your compassion and tolerance grows for yourself and others.

Judgment and blame are the real killers. When we look at life as black and white, right and wrong, we approach people and situations looking for the good guys and the bad guys. In turn, this means that we are either defending ourselves or putting someone else on the defensive.

Our minds are like intricate computers, collecting and processing information. We need to form opinions; it's human nature. But judgment is more than an opinion and it's dangerously limiting.

Judgment is like a locked box. Once we have judged someone or something, we've essentially shut ourselves away from any further opportunity to learn or grow in that situation. When we leave ourselves open (not blanketing the situation with judgment), we are allowing ourselves to expand our awareness. This gives "them" and "us" room to grow. More specifically it's almost impossible to change when someone has a spotlight on your pain: "Your error! Your mistake!"

I don't know anyone who enjoys being judged harshly, or even slightly for that matter. Judgment is focusing on the negative.

Judging yourself too harshly can be crippling. I find it's often easier to forgive others their trespasses than to forgive myself.

Each time you make a judgment, take a moment to evaluate why. Just try to remember that we all need to make mistakes in order to grow. Pain is our teacher. Forgive others and yourself for the need to make mistakes in order to learn. It will give you peace.

Overcoming Negative Thought Patterns and Limited Thinking

If our dreams are contingent on our ability to change someone else's thinking, then we may be waiting a lifetime for our happiness.

More than once I've fallen into that trap, believing that if I could just bring that person around to my way of thinking, everything would be perfect. The assumption that we can change someone else to suit our needs is an exercise in futility.

We're all very complexly and individually created. Hypothetically, I think of myself and others as magnificent patchwork quilts. From the moment we're born, we begin weaving together the threads of our feeling, experiences, and dreams into the intricate patterns that represent who we are.

Usually, it takes years to decipher the crux of the elaborate patterns we weave for ourselves, and even longer to understand the makeup of others.

Sadly, so often during an initial meeting with someone we seem to like, we focus only on those components that may fulfill our needs, rather than appreciate the sum-total picture of who they really are.

What I've done in the past is compromise what I really wanted for what was available at the moment. Upon finding someone who possessed several qualities that I desired but lacked others, I'd simply ignore the problem areas. I'd convince myself that in time I'd change the parts I didn't like.

Until we can wholeheartedly accept that we are entitled to our "perfect" relationship, it's easy to fall prey to our insecurities. I used to spend a great deal of energy trying to convince myself that I could either teach people to see things my way, or conclude that a given issue really wasn't all that important.

In a relationship, as time progresses, people expose who they really are, rather than who we want them to be. Eventually, we begin saying, "Why isn't it as nice as it used to be? Why aren't you like you were? We were happier before."

In reality they were always the same. We had our hopes and dreams, the vision of who we wanted them to be.

Whenever someone else holds the key to our happiness, we have given it to him or her. We have given someone else the responsibility of making us happy.

We can't change people unless they want to be changed. When another person is the object of our problems, then we are the victims, waiting for them to give us what we need. In other words, we must learn to take the emphasis off the *object* of our problems: the person—son, daughter, parent, spouse, or friend. We cannot change people. However, we can change our *perception* of the problem.

When we realize that our *desire* is really the problem, then we have options. If a person is a problem for us, and we desire that they give us something, or change in some way, then *we* have put them in that power position.

Remember, *you are in charge of your perceptions.* But you're not in charge of people.

Fear and insecurity can lead us into the wrong relationship faster than love. It's important to know what our fears are before looking for a partner. After my second divorce, I told myself that I wasn't going to let my fear of being alone influence me in selecting a partner.

Whether it's an obvious conscious fear, or a hidden subconscious one, being afraid of loneliness can color our view of people. It's another way we deceive ourselves by saying, "I can adjust." Thinking that we can change someone just doesn't work in the long run.

While I was trying to find the courage to go it alone, some of my inner dialogue was absolutely terrifying. I told myself negative things like, You're not young anymore, you know. Your career may be over . . . After all, you peaked out in "The Big Valley" eight years ago. And don't forget, you're accustomed to living well. Do you really think you can adapt to being poor again? And maybe there's not going to be a man out there who's right for you. You've already had two marriages that didn't work. Everyone says that the available men are looking for younger women, right?

Fortunately, my belief that I'm entitled to love, happiness, and abundance finally allowed me to overcome those frightening inner voices. I simply changed my inner dialogue to, Okay, Linda, you believe in God. And you're constantly telling people about faith and positive thinking. Well, it's time to practice it yourself. Practice it to the point of facing your fears directly, by going out into the world alone, and proving that it all works.

I quickly learned how important the experience of being alone really is. If only for a day or a weekend, being alone with your thoughts can be a powerful, enlightening experience. A time to learn, reminisce and uncover the old programming, so that you can plan for the new.

Impatience is one of the biggest obstacles we have to overcome. It can be human nature to panic when things are intangible, when we don't have what we want safely in our hands. There have been times when I've felt as though terror and courage were walking hand in hand toward unknown ground.

When I began to learn and understand myself better, trying new methods of analyzing situations, I was desperately impatient, wanting immediate change. Slowly, the process *itself* started becoming absolutely wondrous to me. The journey is really the exciting part, not just the arrival. The point is to enjoy the process, too. Once we learn to trust that we are going in the *right* direction, toward our goals, despite any seemingly *wrong* appearances, we can begin to fully enjoy the journey. The end result will come whether we're impatient or not.

So often we limit our growth, because we limit our thinking; we put mental limitations on our goals. Usually, the only thing standing between me and what I want is all in my thinking. Negative or fearful thoughts can hamper or keep us from our goals and dreams.

I've heard so many people say, "Well, I'm just not as lucky

as the next guy; I don't get the breaks in life." Whether you verbalize it or merely run it through your mind, that kind of limited thinking can stifle your progress.

To some people being rich constitutes being "luckier than others." Many people are born with monetary and material security handed to them. I think being born with money is having one obstacle out of the way. But I've never met anyone who didn't have his own share of lessons to learn and fears to overcome.

Rich or poor, we're all here to learn and grow, and our thinking can either help us or hinder us.

If we allow ourselves to think that we don't deserve the best, or if we believe that we must settle for less than what we want, then how can we reach our full potential?

What I do with negative thoughts is combat them with positive ones. I reverse the thought. In the beginning, changing a thought takes some discipline. It's as though you were teaching yourself a new game: a mind game. It's called, "Fake it until you can make it."

Even if you have to pretend to be positive and happy to get started, anything's better than being unhappy.

I've always been a positive thinker, so this method is obviously easier for me than for someone who leans toward the negative. I've seen this simple process work miraculously on skeptical, negative people. Adults who had been extremely unhappy and depressed since childhood were able to reverse their negative thinking to a generally positive outlook on life; and in the process, everything changed—and improved. Everything!

I watched my step-daughter, Sean, go through this changing process when she was already in her twenties, and very settled in her thinking. As a result of childhood fears and programming, she was locked into perpetual negative thinking patterns. Fortunately, she was willing to give this method of "pretending" a try. Once she'd agreed to experiment, I knew that she could overcome her negativism.

When Sean first started "pretending to be happy," she told me that "It feels very unnatural, and makes me feel very self-conscious to be smiling and laughing so much." However, within just a few days, the positive results and effects started to appear; people were actually responding to her differently, she said. They showed her more warmth and gave her more time and attention than she'd been accustomed to.

It eventually became second nature for her to be positive, even in the face of "negative situations." Progressively, the pretending stopped; she'd adopted a generally positive outlook, because it "felt *right* to be happy." It improved her relationships, career, and above all her sense of self-worth.

We can all change our thinking, if we *believe* it and give it a *try*.

Our Inner Strength/Our Power

"So many people equate strength with possible violation." Patricia explained *power* to me. "If you feel that someone is stronger than you, it may mean that you think they have power over you—power to harm you in some way.

"When we realize that power-over is different from power-of-self authentically expressed, then we are on the way to discerning how to use our strength. Built into this realization is the fact that power-over doesn't work to get you what you really want.

"What we tend to do is create a self-fulfilling prophecy, by defensive maneuvers, and we are the ones harming, and setting ourselves up to be harmed. All the cruelty that *anyone* has ever committed is sourced by an unkind lie that they are believing at the time about themselves, and that is: that they are powerless.

"The power of the self authentically expressed has the strength and earnestness of the truth."

I believe that most of the problems women have with properly exercising their strength stems from centuries of programming: *Woman is the peace maker, the symbol of beauty and harmony; loving, submissive, and passive. Man is the soldier; aggressive, assertive, and strong.*

To varying degrees, our culture has created certain molds to which both men and women are expected to conform. In many cases little girls are told, "Now, you mustn't be overpowering or aggressive. It's very masculine to be assertive." And of course it can be very unattractive when there's no balance, or when strength is expressed solely as a defense mechanism. If it's used just to cover up insecurities, then it's just the illusion of strength, anyway.

Many of us associate strength with masculine energy, and sometimes even violence, simply because for some, that is the experience they've encountered with masculine energy. It's not necessarily only childhood programming, but something that had to be dealt with in adulthood. For example, television popularizes that theory every hour of every day, coupled with true-to-life violent crimes headlining our newspapers continuously.

My learning process involved overcoming my fears of being a strong female. On the other hand, many of my friends had the opposite problem. They needed to express a balance between strength and vulnerability, too, but in order for them to protect their sensitivity, they felt the need to build a defensive wall around them. They were usually terribly bright, and had learned very young to put people off with clever words, or an aggressive manner.

Obviously, people are capable of teaching themselves how to use their intellects to cover up their sensitivity. We can also teach ourselves to stifle our feelings (to some degree), and hold back our opinions. Attack or submit, aggression or passiveness, it's something that we taught ourselves to do, believing at the time that it could keep us safe. What we teach ourselves as children and even as adults is not carved in stone. We alone created our truth and our patterns. Naturally, it stems from something that was very valid to us at the time. But we have the power, the ability to change, if we want to.

What I've learned from my own actions and from my friends' is that there really is a happy medium, a perfect balance in the center between our sensitivity and our strength.

In order to achieve the balance we must first begin to have an earnest appreciation of both sides of our nature.

Begin watching yourself during your interactions with people. If you're reacting from a defensive position, then consciously acknowledge (to yourself) that you're intellectually defending yourself before you're even hurt or threatened. Understand that what you're doing is making it absolutely impossible for you to connect with the best parts of the other person. Be aware that he or she can't really communicate with you through your intellectual shield.

The real key, the most essential part of the process, is to recognize the importance of softness as a force, as a power that is capable of transforming people and situations far better than intellectual defensive aggression.

Meditation

Imagine, if you will, a child's train set. The toy locomotive is going around the track. Everything is running smoothly. Then the dog comes in and sniffs the train, bumping it slightly off its course. Big deal. The train is just a *little* off the rails, but still it doesn't move. The child comes along and wants to play with the train. But it's off the track and it doesn't work. So the child picks it up and smashes it against the wall. Now the train is a whole lot off the track.

The moral of the story? It doesn't matter if your train is a little off or a whole lot off its track. If it's off, it doesn't run.

You must get yourself back on track. And meditation is the best way I know of to do it.

Learning to meditate changed my life. It's the road that leads me to my source and enables me to cope with painful and difficult experiences. Through meditation I've been able to find the inner balance and peace of mind that's so essential during confusing and emotional periods. When I meditate, I become aware of "the lovingness that Created me."

My daily meditations really do help to keep me on the track.

A little over eleven years ago, I did a guest appearance on a television show called, "McCloud." During the filming, Dennis Weaver recommended a book by Paramahansa Yogananda entitled, *An Autobiography of a Yogi.* Because of that book and others I'd read, I was strongly motivated to learn how to meditate. Since then I've studied many of the different techniques available. I began with the methods Paramahansa Yogananda suggested, then read countless books on the subject, including *Transcendental Meditation.* And finally with the help of a dear friend, Reverend Jackie Sorensen, I've learned some unpublicized, easy-to-use techniques, which we will share with you.

Before I actually explain about the meditation, I'd like to tell you a little about the process I went through in the beginning. I suspect there are very few people who can sit down for the first time and go into a blissful meditation.

Originally when I tried to meditate, I'd find a quiet place and sit in a chair with a clock at my side. I'd close my eyes and immediately thoughts started coming into my mind like uncontrollable gusts of wind.

Don't think! I'd say to myself. We're supposed to be meditating. Be quiet!

Within a few minutes, I'd become frantic from all my thoughts running wild. Then, finally when I'd find a moment's silence, I'd think, Oh, great! This is it. Yes, this is what it's supposed to feel like . . . I really think this is it.

Naturally, my enthusiasm immediately disrupted the silence.

Also, when I was sure I'd been sitting there for at least twenty minutes, I'd think, I'll just peek at the clock. Usually, I'd see that only five or ten minutes had elapsed.

Regardless of which meditation technique you choose, you may find that, in the beginning, your thoughts are distracting you. This is simply because we rarely give a voice to anything but our minds, and it's very important for our minds to relinquish total control over us. You're asking your mind to step aside and let your intuitive self speak. Both are important. The information you'll receive (mentally) may be important; listen to it and process it. It may take a week of twenty-minute meditations to process all the old thoughts.

Ultimately, you have power over your thoughts. Think of them as though they were a team of wild horses. They run totally free in every direction if you permit them to. But you have hold of the reins, and can control them, when you're ready.

Meditation is not self-hypnosis. These are two totally and completely different states of mind, and they aren't used to get the same results.

Meditation has been scientifically tested and medically proven to be extremely beneficial for our mental and physical health. Doctors and scientists at accredited universities and laboratories have been able to verify its attributes. For example, meditation (tested under the title of transcendental meditation) proved to: "Decrease blood pressure in hypertensive patients, increase perceptual awareness, decrease anxiety, speed up reaction times, improve performances in job and school, reduce [the use of] alcohol, cigarettes, and nonprescription drugs, and reduce depression and neuroticism." The list of proven benefits goes on and on.

I have asked my dear friend to help me with this section. Reverend Jackie Sorensen is a Minister and Practitioner for The United Church of Religious Science. Together we have devised some exercises and methods to help you enter into meditation. We hope this simplifies the process for you.

Always remember that there are no hard and fast rules to meditating. You have to experiment to see what works best for you. Meditation is a totally personal experience. You are communicating with your innermost self. Everyone is in a "different place," their own unique state of mind, when they sit down to meditate.

HOW TO MEDITATE

When I meditate, I either sit in a chair with my back very straight, or I lie on the floor, couch, or bed with my knees bent up. (I bend my knees when lying down because it prevents my lower back from curving.)

When sitting, I gently rest my hands in my lap, palms up. When lying down, I rest my hands at my sides, also palms up.

I meditate once or twice every day for twenty mintues each time. (Now my twenty minutes fly by!)

In order to meditate you must be relaxed. Reverend Jackie introduced me to an exercise that works very well to prepare for meditation. It goes as follows:

Lie or sit down and become physically comfortable. Then give these instructions (mentally) to your body:

My toes are relaxed. Tense the toes, and then consciously relax them.

My feet are relaxed. Tense the feet, then relax them.

My ankles are relaxed. Tense the ankles, and consciously relax them.

My calves are relaxed. Tense the calves, then relax them.

My thighs are relaxed. Tense the thighs, and consciously relax them.

My hands are relaxed. Tense the hands, then relax them.

My arms are relaxed. Tense the arms, and then relax them.

My shoulders are relaxed. Tense the shoulders, and relax them.

I now relax all the muscles in my neck so that my head falls quite free. All the tension leaves my head and my face. My temples are relaxed, my eyelids and my unclenched jaw are totally relaxed.

I'm in a complete state of relaxation, from my head to my toes.

BREATHING INTO MEDITATION

Deep-breathing exercises are a wonderful, easy way to get into meditation.

Simply make yourself physically comfortable and close your eyes. Exhale!

Take a deep breath in through your nose. Blow out the air through your mouth.

Breathe deeply and slowly.

As you inhale and exhale, count your breaths (mentally). *One,* as you inhale. *Two,* as you exhale. *Three, four, five,* and so on.

Concentrate only on your breathing and counting.

Should you lose track of the count, as a result of a thought coming to mind, simply begin at *one* again. You don't have to fight your thoughts, just count over them.

Breathe in and out slowly until you are completely and perfectly relaxed.

OTHER WAYS TO ENTER MEDITATION

When thoughts are continuously interrupting your silence, one of the best ways to overcome them is to use a *mantra*. A mantra is a Hinduism. It is used as in incantation to replace the thoughts with a pleasant-sounding word. For example: Peace, love, and om are commonly used as mantras. What a great many people do is chant "om," almost singing it. You would take a deep breath and, stretching the syllables, as you exhale say, 'Oooohmmmmmm" (it may sound a little silly to you at first, but it actually feels lovely once you get accustomed to it).

Any word that pleases your mind's ear will work. Simply repeat the word over and over and over in your mind (or aloud if you prefer). Gently, very smoothly and softly. Every time a thought sneaks in, just say a word over them, until the peace, the silence is resumed.

You may find that the first few times you try meditating you'll drift off to sleep, it's so relaxing. It's okay. It usually means that you're just tired.

If you find that your thoughts are just too distracting, even after you've done the physical exercise, the breathing, and the mantra, there's yet another valid way to reach a state of meditation.

If anxiety or pressing problems are too distracting, I suggest that you use the following *visualization exercises* to release your fears before meditating. You might find it quite helpful to put the exercises on tape and play them back when you're ready to spend the time to relax, release, and meditate. If you don't particularly enjoy hearing yourself on tape (as many don't), then find someone whose voice you do find soothing.

For example: Making yourself physically comfortable, breathe deeply and close your eyes. Relax!

Imagine you're on the bank of a glorious flowing river. Visualize it, as only you can. See the blue sky reflected on the shimmering currents.

Breathe in and really smell nature's beauty around you. All your favorite trees and flowers are within your reach.

You hear only the sounds you adore. Be it birds, the water rustling, or the wind in the trees, hear it, really hear it.

Then you move gracefully to the edge of the water. Holding tight to a beautiful tree beside you, you put your toes into the river.

The current suddenly tries to pull you into its flow, but you cling desperately to the tree, deeply fearing the unknown waters.

Suddenly you realize that you want to *let go*. You really want to give in to the natural flow and you release your fearful grip, trusting that life will carry you on the right course.

You're flowing with the river, beholding the splendor above and around you.

You are completely relaxed and confident.

When the river leads you to a fork, you know that you will take the right direction, you are so free of fear and anxiety.

As you close your eyes, visualize yourself walking on the beach. Feel the cool sand under your feet, the warm sun on your back, the salt spray moist on your face.

After a while, you move into the water. It feels wonderful; the temperature is ideal for you.

Feel yourself becoming part of a wave, moving up and down rhythmically. Soon you are the wave, you have melted into it and feel completely relaxed. All the tension is gone, you're totally free. You can hear the sounds of the ocean. Listen to them and become one with them.

Relax, and hear only the silence.

Become physically comfortable, close your eyes and you're walking through a tropical forest. Visualize the trees and the animals around you. Hear the sounds, smell the freshness. Everything is alive, awake, and serene. It's a beautiful experience for you.

You're on a path that leads you to a picturesque, tranquil lake. Water lillies are on the surface, and reeds sprout at the edge. The water is as clean and calm as glass, until an occasional fish splashes by.

As you gaze into the still waters you feel your oneness with all life.

Remain there as long as you like. You're relaxed and content as the silence begins.

Become physically comfortable.

The only thing you hear is the sound of your breathing. Listen, really concentrate on it. Breathe deeply and rhythmically.

Slowly begin to mentally visualize a large, brightly colored *ball* of light glowing above you. The ball starts to grow bigger and bigger. Keep seeing it grow until it's all-consuming. Then when you're ready, watch it slowly shrink. The ball shrinks into a mere speck and finally disappears into nothing at all.

Now do the same exercise, but this time fill the floating ball with all your pain. As you add your pain to it, see it become bigger and bigger, until *all* your pain is in the ball.

Then when the ball is full, make a decision as to whether you want to keep the pain in your life or let it go.

If you're ready to release it, if you don't want it anymore, then see the ball begin to shrink. Actually visualize it floating higher and higher, farther and farther away until it is a speck in the sky, and finally it's gone completely.

Then relax, knowing you are free. Listen to the silence.

A Very Special Section

Because of my natural curiosity and insatiable appetite for knowledge and self-improvement, I have studied many of the popular and more obscure ancient sciences. Astrology, numerology, I Ching, and tarot are some of the tools that can help you get in touch with your intuition. When they're understood and applied properly, they can be invaluable.

Having invested a great deal of time studying and working with these sciences, I know firsthand many of their benefits and limitations. I have been taught by experts in all these fields, participating both as a paying client and as a friend. I've also been a practicing numerologist for well over ten years.

In today's society, investigating astrology, meditation, or any of the other alternatives that help you develop your intuitive sense is more acceptable than ever before. Many intelligent, logical people acknowledge that these are excellent methods for enlightenment as well as legitimate sources of information.

One of the limitations I've encountered in my pursuit of enlightenment is a tendency to become dependent on astrologers, psychics, or anyone who seems to have "The Answer." When we allow ourselves to become dependent on someone else's assessment of what's best for us, we have given up our *free will,* and given someone else power—over us.

It's very helpful to find out as much as you can about the person you're going to see. Whether it's an astrologer, or psychic, it's important to know how they utilize their power. The question is, do they make you more aware of your abilities, or merely feed you destructive information. The best way to determine how someone works is to ask the person recommending them, "How did you feel after the reading? Enlightened, or full of fear and doubts?"

Remember, *astrology is not the answer to our problems, it is merely a wonderful tool.* It can be an enjoyable, productive way to shed some light on our personal patterns and dramas. I've always been fascinated and intrigued by astrology because it helps me to better understand myself and others.

Linda McCallum, introduced earlier, a highly intuitive astrologer, has taught me a great deal over the last several years. *Even* Linda, an accredited, professional astrologer, doesn't refer daily to her astrology books. It simply gives her an excellent idea of what the options may be.

Professionally, Linda uses astrology as a practical means of uncovering psychological patterns and freeing people to utilize their power. One of the advantages of a complete chart is that it can accurately describe our earlier environment and conditioning, including parts of our childhood that we have blocked or forgotten. Astrology can give you basic insights into all areas of your life: your partnerships, work, career, sex, love, and children. It uncovers both your aptitudes and the places where you've accepted limitations.

The key is always to remember: Astrology is merely an insight.

OUR INTUITIVE SENSE

I'm certain that we are all born with an intuitive awareness, a special ability to comprehend above and beyond that which is apparent. We usually dismiss the inexplicable feeling connected with our *gut instincts,* our intuitive sense, because we can't find a way to intellectually justify them. Our rational minds want information that's more tangible, more scientific to process. Unfortunately, we don't normally allow ourselves the freedom to openly trust this "instinctual" part of ourselves.

Since I've permitted myself to readily acknowledge these *gut* feelings my life has greatly improved. We *all* have this valuable asset at our disposal. But we must learn to develop it.

Nine years ago I went to see a highly recommended pyschic therapist named Jacqueline Eastlund. Jackie is a very loving, spiritual, and intuitive woman. We have been close friends ever since my initial pyschic reading. I asked Jackie if she'd help me to explain how one should go about choosing a suitable pyschic (if so desired) and how *we* can learn to develop our intuitive sense. I'm very happy that Jackie agreed to share her views with us.

Jackie strongly believes that we should never go to a clairvoyant, or psychic, unless he or she has been highly recommended by someone we trust implicitly.

It is also very important to understand that there is no one on earth who is one hundred percent accurate at reading the future. Only God has that magnitude of power. But a legitimate, qualified psychic should be able to tell you at *least* a little bit of your past with relative accuracy. It is not unreasonable to request that they read something of your past before going into your future. If they blatantly botch up this initial test, then it is reasonable to assume that they will also fail to see what's in store for your future.

Once you've established a comfortable rapport with a psychic, it's imperative that you don't lose sight of your free will. E.S.P. is just another insight, not the answer to our problems.

Everyone has E.S.P. For the most part people believe that they don't need it to survive, and have consequently sadly neglected it. Even so, at some point in our lives, we all experience different degrees of E.S.P.: a mother's sense of her child's well-being, thinking about a friend minutes before she phones, or suddenly deciding to turn down a street and finding you've avoided an accident. There are dozens of unexplained reactions that relate to our intuitive sense. And although more often than not we simply ignore our intuition during our waking hours, while we're asleep, it's busy sending us information in our dream state. Many people find it useful to keep a special book to record their dreams, because they realize that it's their subconscious mind advising them.

Jackie has helped me and many of my friends to heighten our intuitive awareness. It takes patience, discipline and a commitment. But if you're seriously interested in developing your intuitive sixth sense, a healthy mind and body are important. Drugs and alcohol often interfere with our mental balance, so they should be avoided.

We feel the easiest way to begin developing your sixth sense is to concentrate on fine-tuning your other five senses: sight, hearing, touch, taste, and smell.

Think of this learning process as an exercise. In a sense, you are "working out" particular muscles. It can be a very rewarding personal experience.

Begin by going for a walk alone. The purpose is to learn how to concentrate on your individual senses. Try to pay attention to everything around you as though you were taking a walk for the first time in your life. Look at the sky, see the shapes of the clouds. Look around you, see the greens of the trees, observe the houses, the cars, and the flowers.

After a little while sit down and listen. Spend your energy just hearing. Shut your eyes and concentrate on all the sounds around you: the birds, the wind, or the cars.

Don't rush. Enjoy the beauty of it. We take our five senses for granted. Spend five minutes, or as long as you like, just touching. Take a leaf and feel it. Then close your eyes and really sense it. Feel the veins, the different textures; some are smooth and others rough. Become aware of the differences.

Again, keeping your eyes shut, gently taste your skin. You may immediately have a mental picture of salt. Whatever you taste, spend some time concentrating on how your mouth is reacting to it.

Later, find a flower or a blade of grass, something pleasant smelling, and concentrate on it. Using only your sense of smell, be aware of the difference in the fragrances.

After you have taken time to enjoy these personal moments exercising your five senses, find a quiet place where you can sit down and write down everything you recall about the experience. Keep a special notebook handy to record and date all the thoughts and feelings you receive. After writing this down, take the same walk again and see what you missed the first time. You'll be amazed. You'll see that we don't really pay attention to what we perceive through our five senses. This is an excellent way to teach yourself concentration.

These particular sense exercises will help you increase your overall awareness. They will aid you in becoming more sensitive and in touch with parts of yourself that normally function automatically. Remember, our sixth sense also functions all the time, but if we are not in tune to it, it is of little use to us.

One of the best ways to receive sixth-sense information is during meditation. You may want to try one of the meditations I use. (See pages 39–43.) As I've said, I meditate every day because it enables me to become balanced and relaxed. My daily meditation is designed to center myself. When I am working specifically with my intuitive sense, I will take a separate half-hour meditation. Jackie suggests simply repeating the word *love* over and over, gently, in your mind, while entering a state of meditation.

Once you have cleared your mind through twenty minutes of meditation, you can then practice your intuitive perception on anything you like. For example, you can concentrate on a particular object. Take any object that is not washed and gently hold it in the palms of your hands. Sit very still with your eyes closed and "see" if you can sense or envision anything.

Concentrating on a particular friend is another helpful exercise. See if you can sense what he or she is doing. Then check later to see if you sensed correctly.

Another single exercise you can do with a deck of regular playing cards: Take one card at a time (face down) from the pile and place your hand over it with your eyes closed. Then concentrate on the color. Black or red? Then turn it over and see if you guessed right. Keep score of how many you guessed correctly. After you get seventy percent right, try sensing the suit.

Try to practice at least one of the suggested methods for thirty minutes a day. Remember to write down any thoughts you perceived during your sense exercises, meditations, or object practices.

As your intuition increases, you'll also begin to receive psychic data when you are not consciously concentrating on it. Perhaps this will occur when you are driving along quietly, or just before you go to sleep. Anytime you have a flash, or a feeling, try to remember it long enough to write it down. That way you will have a diary of your progression. You will be able to refer to it when things begin to happen as you *sensed* they would.

These are only a few ways Jackie and I suggest you begin. However, the most important thing to remember is you *do* already have extrasensory perception. (It will reveal itself when you are able to accept it.) Pay attention to that still small voice within. It is an important part of *you.*

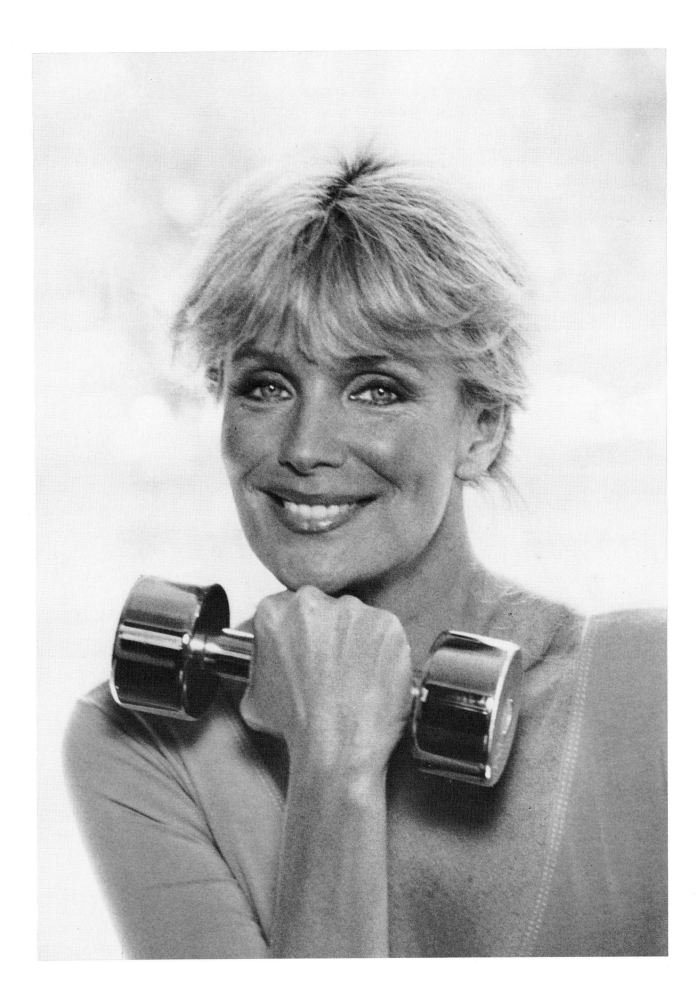

PART TWO

OUTER BEAUTY

An Introduction to Outer Beauty

Where shall you seek beauty, and how shall you find her unless she herself be your way and your guide?
—*The Prophet,*
Kahlil Gibran

Over the years a lot of people have said to me, "I just can't believe how much you've changed." Usually, they'd have come across an old photograph or a rerun of "The Big Valley" television series, and noticed that my face had been heavier, my hair was different, and, although I've always been thin, my general muscle tone wasn't as it is today. People are constantly asking me, "How were you able to change?"

Looking the very best that I can helps me to feel positive about myself, while staying in shape and keeping healthy gives me the freedom to take my mind off myself, and enables me to concentrate on the important things in life.

There are certainly enough trying experiences to go through, to absorb and comprehend, without having our bodies as an obstacle.

We don't have to settle for what we don't like about the way we look. We have so many options available to us today: makeup, massage, hair styles, facials, exercise, and, if you choose, plastic surgery.

The first step is to stand in front of your mirror and see what you have to work with. Ask yourself honestly, "What do I like about myself? What are my biggest assets? What really bothers me the most about my appearance? What would I like to change? Is my hair style really right for me? Am I using the right makeup for my face and is it improving my looks?

"And what about my body? How can I improve on my figure? Where do I need to build up and where should I trim down?"

One thing's for sure, if you don't give yourself a chance, nothing will happen.

There are dozens of ways to get into shape, to improve the way you look and how you feel. But before anything can change, you have to make a commitment to yourself. And most of all you have to want the end results.

Aging Shouldn't Mean Falling Apart

With the ancient is wisdom;
and in length of days
understanding.
    —Old Testament; Job 12:12

Unfortunately, our society is geared toward accepting that as people grow older, they are not as valuable; consequently, their lives are less meaningful. I fully believe the opposite to be true.

The most important thing to remember is that you don't have to "fall apart" and look terrible just because you're getting older. However, if you accept that in your thirties, or with "middle age," you'll begin to fall apart, then you probably will. If you set new goals for yourself, if you say to yourself, I'm not going to let myself go until I'm eighty-five; there's no reason I should give up. No matter what anyone says! I have control over the situation. Then you have a long-range positive plan for retaining (loving) your face and body, not destroying them.

Lola's Facial Techniques

I've known Lola for many years now. She does, as she puts it, "facial rejuvenation and recontouring." I asked her to explain how the facial technique works, before actually going into how you can apply it to yourself.

As a result of Lola's facials, my skin actually looks better, "younger" than before. The theory, the technique, was discovered nearly fifty years ago by two doctors and a cosmetologist. It works for me, as people have noticed and commented. And many of my friends have had the same positive results.

Lola has consented to share the technique and has also given us easy-to-use methods for everyday do-it-yourself facial exercises and cleaning.

The muscles in the face usually begin to sag when we are about twenty-five: slowly, gently, and imperceptibly, like earth eroding. What happens, more often than not, is that we look in the mirror one day and it seems as though our face has begun to sag quite suddenly. Actually it was a slow process.

The two doctors and the cosmetologist who taught Lola evolved a method of correctly and validly exercising the nineteen muscles in the face which keep the skin from sagging. What the exercise does is put the muscles under tension and flush extra blood through them.

In this technique, a far greater amount of blood than is normally carried through the face is pumped up by way of manipulating or massaging the muscles on either side of the neck. (This treatment can only be given by those practitioners who have been specially trained.) This extra blood is brought up to the face by the arterial system. Then it begins to drain down the face by the vascular system on its way back to the heart. As the blood is draining down the face Lola catches (manipulates) the facial muscles and puts them under very precise tension, thus flushing the extra blood through the muscles. This tightens, tones, and exercises the muscles throughout the entire facial treatment. She keeps going back and massaging up more blood to work with. The skin cells (in the face) die and then reproduce three times faster than the cells in the body. After each facial treatment Lola does for me, I notice that my face and skin appear tighter and more toned.

When I go to Lola for my facials, she puts me into a complete and total state of relaxation by massaging my neck and upper back and feet. Tension is one of the greatest causes of aging because it blocks the flow of blood to the face. When we are nervous and "knotted up," the blood flow is constricted, and blood is essential for good skin and strong healthy muscles. Unfortunately, Lola is in Malibu, California, (Lola by the Sea) and obviously not everyone can go to her for treatments. However, these simple facial techniques, which she has written out for you, are very helpful and can actually improve your skin.

So that you can work without a facial technician, Lola has suggested the following steps: Once or, if possible, twice a day, get your head lower than your feet, either with pillows or a slant board or a gravity device to encourage blood to rush to the face and scalp (which even encourages hair growth). This would be a good time to do deep breathing or any form of meditation or restful non-thought.

Then a series of hot (not steaming) and cold (not ice cubes) towels can be applied to the face to stir up the circulation. (Intense steam can break the capillaries and strip the skin of the desirable sebaceous oil, which keeps you younger-looking. And ice cubes can also break capillaries.)

To clean the skin in a thorough way (after two or three hot towels applied to the skin) dry both skin and hands and then apply raw, unprocessed honey (Lola and I like Tupolo honey because we think it is also the best for eating). Leave the honey on for two or three minutes to expose it to the air so that it becomes very sticky and then take your fingers and *press in* and *snap out* with the honey (picturing that you are vacuum-cleaning the pores of debris, makeup, etc.). Just *avoid the eye area* from the brow to about three quarters of an inch below the eye because the skin is delicate and its capillaries can break if it is too vigorously snapped with the honey. When the skin has had all oil, creams, or makeup removed, and the pores opened (by way of a couple of hot towels and then dried as are the hands), honey used in this way is one of the best methods of deep-cleaning the pores. (A warm, damp towel will remove the honey.)

When the pores are relieved of impacted material they begin

to shrink and become refined, smaller, and more attractive. Distended pores impacted with dark grease and oil is what you will be working to reverse.

The two face strokes that you can do safely by yourself are these: *the mouth and the cheek stroke.*

Put a bit of cream on your mouth and your fingertips. Firmly but gently pinch the mouth together. Always work from the outside of the mouth area to the inside. Then start again at the outer corners of the mouth and pinch inward. Do this over and over for about five minutes (or during the commercials on your favorite TV show—as a distraction). Remember, don't pinch inward and go outward; always start from the outer part and go in.

The *mouth stroke* used regularly will quickly tighten up the *round muscle* that goes around your mouth. When it sags with age and decreasing estrogen, it causes those little lines around the mouth we all hate that lipstick bleeds up into. They will soften and fade when the round-mouth muscle is tightened. There is another lovely side effect; the lips will get fuller from toning this muscle.

The *second stroke* that you can do with great benefit is the *cheek stroke.* The cheek stroke will help to tighten the muscles that, when allowed to sag, create the unsightly lines from the corner of the nose to the corner of the mouth. Here, with cream on the cheeks and fingers, you stroke firmly *outward. Always outward,* beginning at either side of the nose just under the cheekbone. With index and third finger slide along under the cheekbone. Lean on the cheekbone and don't slide down to the muscle beneath it. End your stroke about an inch in front of the ear. You might alternate between mouth and cheek stroke. Do each about eight times.

The most common misinformation in regard to face massage is that you can stretch the skin in a negative way. This is simply untrue. The only way skin is ever stretched is by way of weight gain, such as in pregnancy.

Lola intimately knows the construction of the muscles so that she can lift and apply tension and exercise them correctly. Those were two that you can safely use for yourself to exercise a portion of the face that tends to age more noticeably.

Also, Lola recommends using witch hazel pads or chamomile tea bags on the eyes. This can help lighten the dark circles under the eyes, and also help to shrink the little lines. Plus, it can be generally soothing and relaxing to the eyes.

The two products you really need, besides a cleanser, are a pure moisturizer and a sunscreen or block. Honey is one very special way of deep-cleaning the pores. But you should remove heavy makeup first with a cleanser, lotion, or soap. Whatever you feel cleans best for you. Remember products with "beauty grains" can be abrasive, giving skin a kind of sandpaper feel and look.

The best thing for skin is *relaxation*, allowing blood to circulate through it naturally, with all its benefits.

A SPECIAL EXERCISE FOR YOUR NECK AND CHIN

Here's a very productive but "funny-looking" exercise to tighten up the muscles under your chin. Try it in front of a mirror, with a side view (profile) of yourself, so you can actually see the benefits.

Open your mouth and stick out your tongue as far as you can, pointing the tip upward. You should see and feel the muscles in your neck tightening up. Do this tongue-in-and-out exercise about twenty-five times in a row to begin. Then each week, add more repetitions as the muscles get stronger. You will quickly see results.

Warning: I suggest you do this exercise privately to avoid ridicule.

Makeup

Armando Cosio has been a professional makeup artist for fifteen years. We have been working together steadily for just over two years now. I first became aware of Armando because I make it a habit to look up the names of makeup artists responsible for the work I admire in magazines. I'm by no means the only face Armando makes up. Elizabeth Taylor, Raquel Welch, Olivia Newton-John, Brooke Shields, Beverly Sassoon, and Victoria Principal are only a handful of the famous faces that Armando works with.

Armando making me up for the photo session with Mario Caselli for the cover of this book.

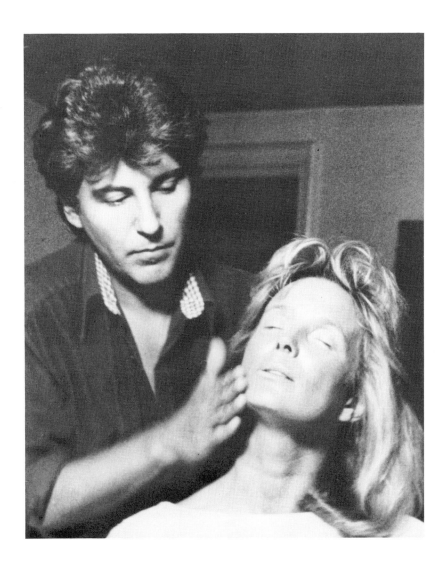

He is in the process of writing his own professional beauty book. However, he has consented to share the makeup tips and methods that he has taught me.

Obviously, makeup for still- and motion-picture photography is different from our normal day and evening needs. Armando has a successful beauty salon in Los Angeles, where he makes up women for both show business and everyday use. The following section on makeup is for day and evening use, not professional photography. It includes what I feel is the most important information I've ever learned about makeup. It works for me.

EYES

It's all in the eyes . . .

One of the most flattering looks for the eyes I've ever seen is a trick that models, on the covers of high-fashion magazines around the world, have used for years.

I've seen it done time and time again, but I could never figure out how they did it. I read all the magazine articles but they always kept that particular part a secret. Then one day, Armando did it to my eyes. After years of frustration, the secret was finally mine. Now it's yours, too.

For this "secret" look, you will need only black cake eyeliner, and a very thin (small) sable brush.

Lift your eyelid slightly to expose the thin rim of skin under lash base. Take the sable brush, dip it into water, and blend a small amount of the black cake eyeliner on it.

Carefully draw a dark line with the brush on the exposed rim close to the lashes. Then immediately put down the brush, still holding your eye open, and carefully fan the wet rim of the eye until the liner is dry. Then lower the lid.

The cake liner keeps the color from smearing down to the bottom rim as most pencils would. This gives you a thicker-looking lash, without a line, for summer at the beach or daytime. It even looks great in the evening with eye shadows and the pencils Armando recommends using around the eyes (found in the following eye section).

When applying certain eye makeup your vision has to be very good, or as Armando pointed out to me, there are special magnifying eye glasses (in which the lenses actually lift up on either side so that you can both see *and* put on your makeup), and of course there are many powerful magnifying mirrors.

To do your eyes you will need: an eyelash curler, black mascara, three eye pencils (thin ones)—brown, gray, and black—gray-brown powder shadow, gray powder shadow, taupe (a brownish-gray) powder shadow, black cake eyeliner, and an eyebrow brush. These shadow colors are fairly neutral and will enhance *any* eye colors.

Line over and under entire eyes with brown pencil very close to the lashes, and blend with fingertips, Q-tip, or a small sable brush. Your eyes should be surrounded with a haze of color, not a heavy dark line.

Now take your taupe powder eyeshadow and brush it over the pencil line to set and to further soften the blended effect. Then take a little taupe shadow and brush it on the eyelids from the lash line to just slightly above the eye crease and blend carefully.

Curl the lashes and apply two coats of black mascara (for recommended mascara application see below).

To further define the eyes you can line the upper and lower inside rim of the eye with gray or brown pencil.

Mascara. Curl the lashes, apply one light coat of mascara and wait a few minutes. Then lift the eyelid slightly to expose the thin rim of skin at the lash base. Now take the tip of the mascara wand and dot mascara carefully at the base of the lashes. Remember, the greatest amount of color and thickness should be at the base of the lashes and not on the tips.

Now brush on more mascara in the normal manner to distribute it to the tips of the lashes.

Applying mascara this way will create the effect of a thicker, darker lash base that beautifully frames the eyes and tapers to a fine feathery tip or end.

Eyebrows. Your eyebrows frame your eyes and also give them expression.

To properly tweeze eyebrows: Soften the brows by saturating two cotton balls or a washcloth in hot water. Place the saturated material over the brows. Allow it to remain long enough to relax and soften the eyebrow tissue.

To remove the hairs from above the eyebrow line: brush hair downward, then shape the upper section.

To remove the hair from under the brow line: brush hair upward and shape the lower section.

Make sure you tweeze all the stray hairs and alternate between both brows to obtain proper balance.

After you have tweezed the brows, carefully wipe the area with an astringent to contract the skin. Then brush the hair, placing it in its normal position. Pencil where necessary.

The high point of the arch should be just above where the iris (the colored part of the eye) meets the white on the outer corner.

A soft lead drawing pencil is best for very dark or black brows.

Taupe eyebrow pencil is best for brown shades.

Silverized beige is best for blondes.

A little hair spray on your eyebrow brush will help control unruly brows and keep them in place.

MOISTURIZER

Another suggestion Armando has given me concerns moisturizing. It's important to treat your neck with the same special care you give to your face. Whenever you cleanse, scrub, or moisturize your face, you should always remember to do the same to your neck. The skin on your neck is very delicate and wrinkles as easily as the face. Whenever possible, also moisturize the skin just behind the ear (unfortunately, it tends to make the hair oily, but it's still part of the face).

Personally, I like to use tinted moisturizers instead of makeup, especially during the summer when I have a slight suntan.

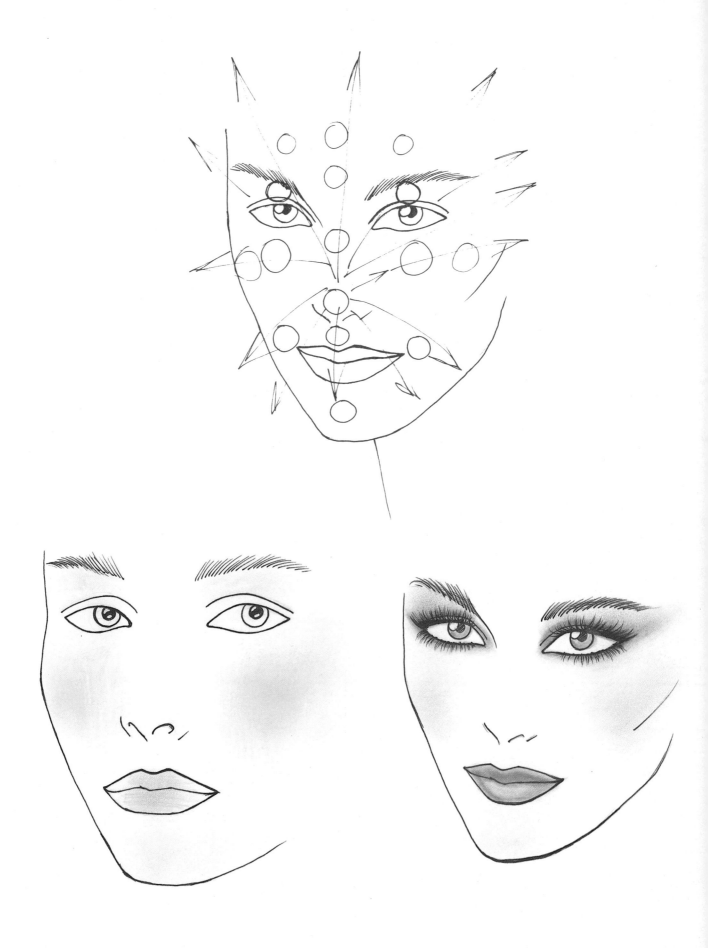

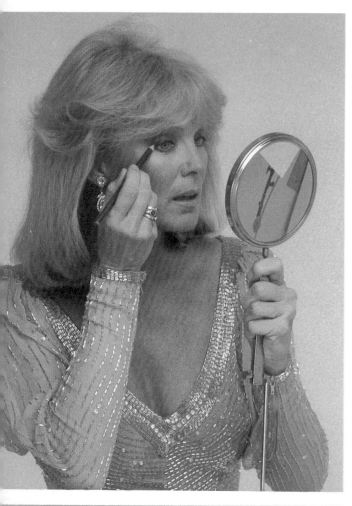

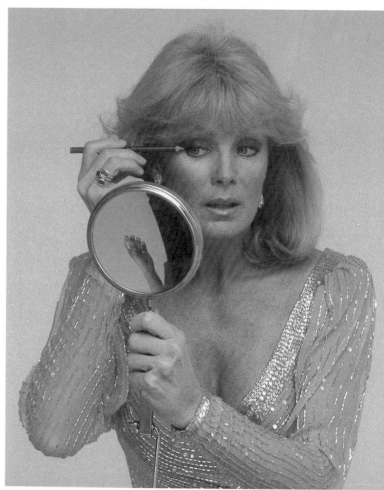

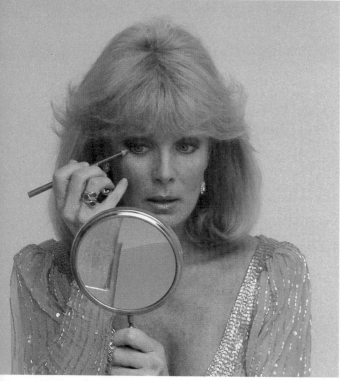

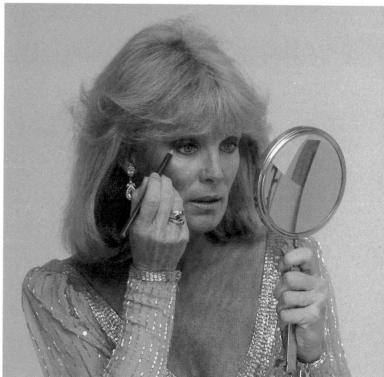

Using a thin brown eye pencil, draw a line over and under the entire eye, very close to the lashes. Blend with fingertip, Q-tip, or small sable brush.

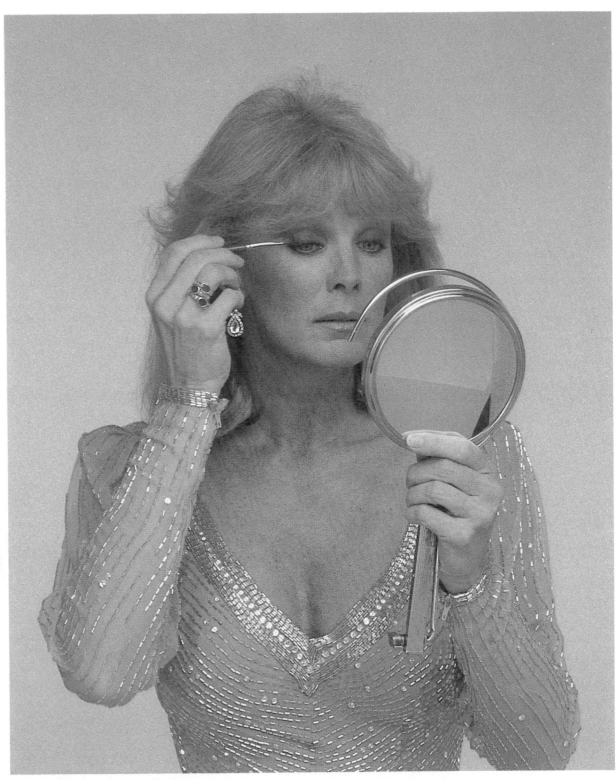

**Brush taupe powder eye shadow
over pencil to set . . .**

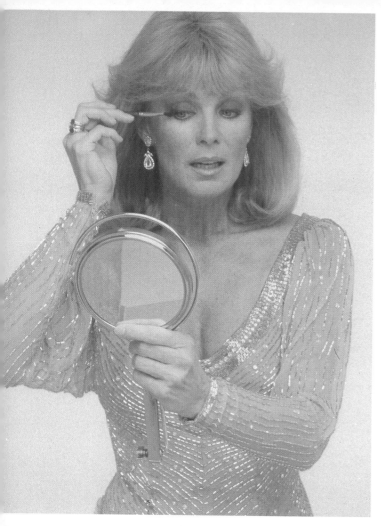

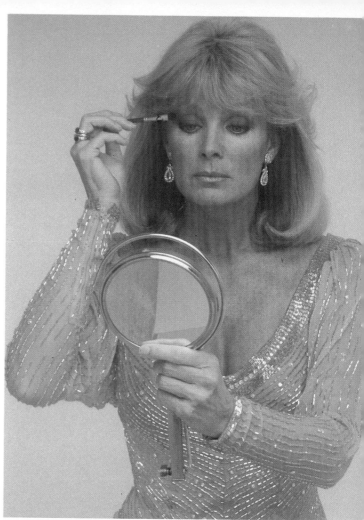

. . . then brush some taupe shadow from lash line to just slightly above eye crease and blend carefully.

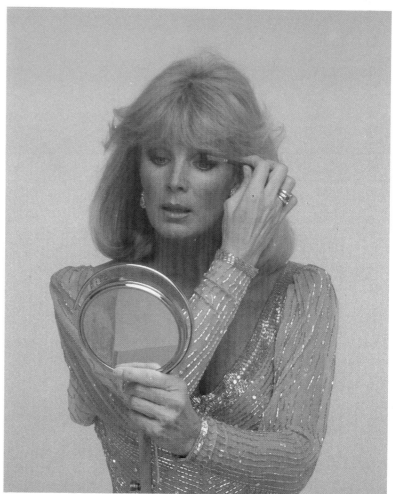

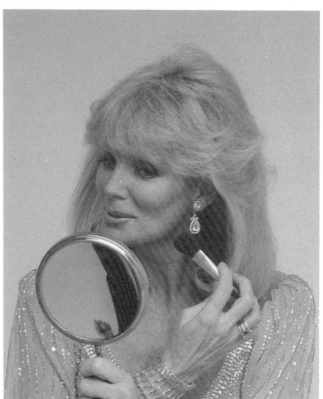

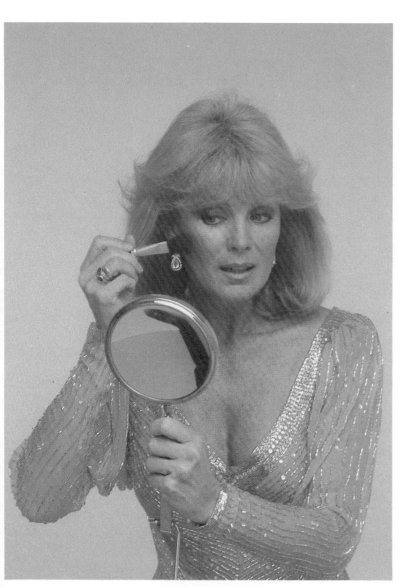

Apply loose translucent powder with a large powder brush to set makeup and reduce shiny areas.

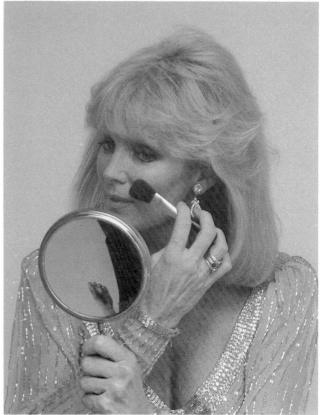

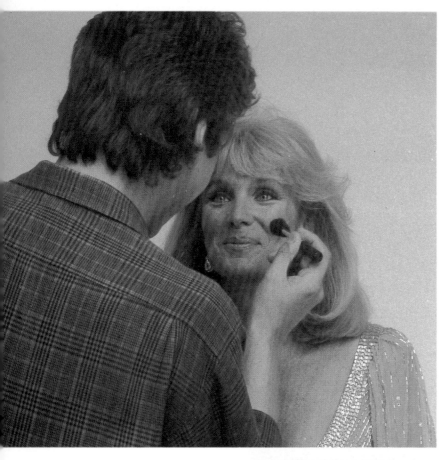

Armando at work . . .

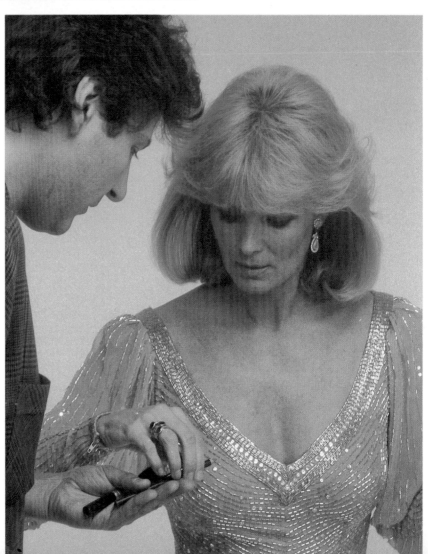

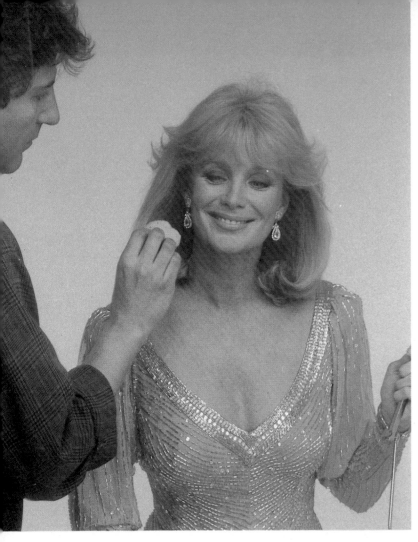

The finishing touches.

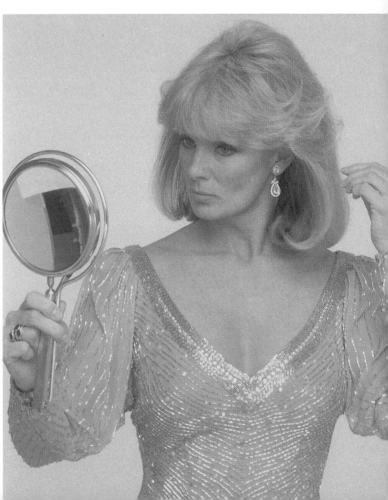

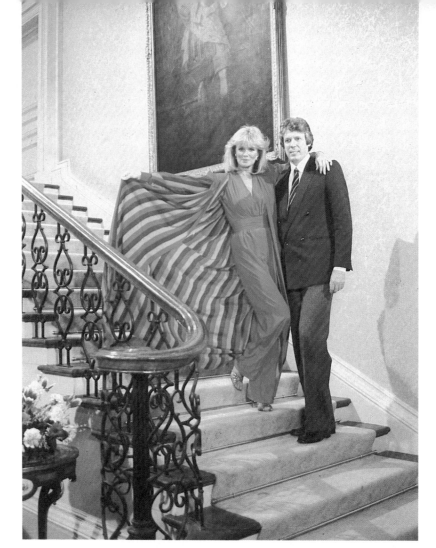

Nolan Miller and I on the set of "Dynasty."

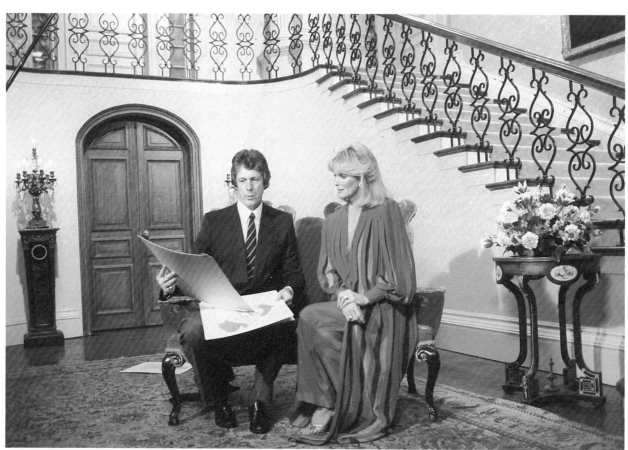

Many women think that the older they get the more makeup they need. Armando has shown me that that's not always the case. As we get older the colors we use are more crucial than when we were younger, but the less makeup applied the younger the face will usually look. Caking on the makeup only accentuates the lines in the face.

FOUNDATION

After your skin has been properly cleansed, toned, and moisturized, wait five to ten minutes for your skin to normalize.

Be sure to select a color that will match your neck color so that you won't have to apply it all the way down your neck (and ruin your expensive clothes). Remember you are trying to *match* your skin tone, not change it.

Dot your foundation on lightly, and concentrate the application in the center of your face.

Four dots on your forehead.

One dot on each eyelid.

One dot under each eye.

One dot on the bridge of the nose.

One dot on the tip of the nose.

One dot on the cheeks.

One dot on the area under the nose and above the lips.

One dot on the outside corners of the mouth.

One dot on the chin. (See page 64)

Now blend with a slightly damp high-quality makeup sponge; from the bridge of your nose upward toward your hairline, then downward over the tip of the nose, upper lip, lips, chin, and jaw.

Then across the bridge of the nose to the inner eye corner, under the eyes and eyelids, and out toward the hairline. Finally, from the nose again, to the cheeks, ear, and jawline.

"Use long, smooth strokes and blend carefully."

Think of a starburst as you blend quickly and evenly.

The effect should be like a drop of watercolor on a wet piece of paper—the most intensity in the center, fading to almost nothing as it reaches the outer perimeter.

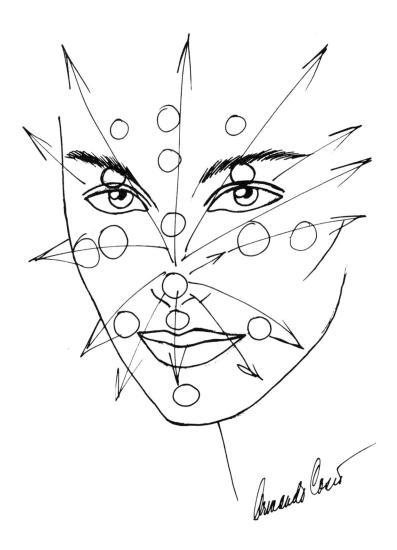

Some women often make the mistake of applying their foundation so heavily that they end up with the makeup collecting at the hairline, on the ears, and at an unsightly demarcation line showing around the jawline.

ROUGE

A light application of cream rouge before powdering is by far the best way to get a lovely natural glow that seems almost as though it's coming from within. It gives the skin a moist, dewey, fresh young look unlike powder blushes that sometimes seem to just sit there on the surface like a coating. (But Armando has a great trick for powder on page 66.)

A special tip: If you don't have cream rouge just use a few dabs of your lipstick. It works beautifully and gives you a lovely glow.

Application of cream rouge (see below). Apply cream rouge with fingertips or a dry latex sponge. Place a dot of rouge on each cheek. Then use what's left on your sponge or fingers and blend on your eyelids, forehead, and then on your chin.

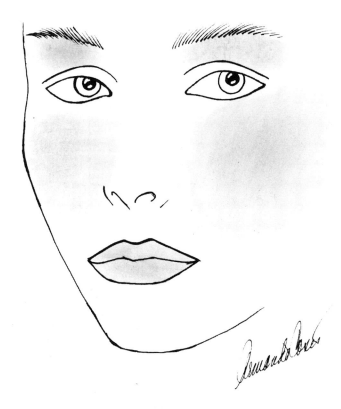

Application of powder blush. If you must wear powder rouge or blush because of skin breakouts from the cream ones, here's a trick that works very well with powder blushes.

After powdering with translucent loose powder (see next section), apply the powder blush layer by layer instead of all at once.

After you've applied the desired amount, take a high-quality makeup sponge that's been dampened with cool water and press lightly over the powdered rouge until all the excess powder has been absorbed by the sponge. Somehow, you get a more translucent, natural look.

POWDER

Use a loose, translucent powder, brushed on with a large powder brush. This will set your makeup, help it last longer, and reduce any shiny areas.

Begin with your forehead, then your nose, eyelids, chin, and finally your neck.

After you've applied the desired amount of powder, take a high-quality makeup sponge that's been dampened with cool water and press gently over the powdered areas until all the excess powder has been absorbed by the sponge. It will give you a

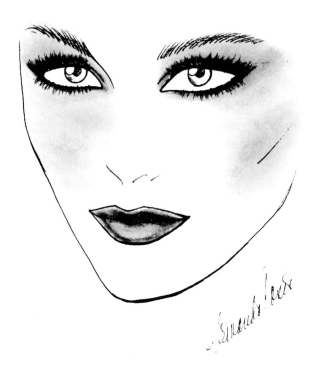

more natural look. This is something I always do after powdering my face.

At this point you may just want to add a little mascara to your already curled lashes. Then a bit of gloss to your lips and you'll have a wonderfully clean, healthy, natural look. (See page 66.)

LIPS

To achieve very natural-looking, beautiful lips, apply your lipstick in the usual manner, and then simply blot until there's only a strain or hint of color left. Then add just a bit of gloss for shine.

If your lips are "too" full, just line them slightly *within* your own natural lip line.

If your lips are "too" thin, line them slightly *outside* your natural lip line.

Always match your lipliner to your lipstick so that you *never* have an obvious outline.

If you're the type of woman who doesn't look well in a lot of lip color, use tinted lip gloss or make your own by using your favorite lipstick and mixing it with clear lip gloss.

If your lip color doesn't last: Apply lipstick, and blot powder slightly over lips, and then reapply lipstick.

CONCEALER OR COVER

Armando usually waits until he's done all the makeup before using any concealer, because once you've emphasized all your features, the imperfections are less noticeable and therefore need minimal attention.

This way you avoid that overly concealed look, like white rings around the eyes, heavy deposits of light pigment around the nostrils, mouth, and eyes. You don't want your coverups competing with your eyes, lips, or cheeks, thereby defeating your prime purpose.

Nail Care

A few years ago I went to Teressa Reno, seeking help for my nails. She had been highly recommended by a good friend of mine. I was upset over the condition of my nails and tired of hearing, "It could be health or lack of proper vitamins." It was disheartening to spend time and money only to end up with peeling nails and frayed cuticles a day after the manicure.

Reno told me that the health of my nails was perfect. She added that I could have beautiful nails. I was curious about that statement. I asked her what she could do that was different. Here is a short résumé on nails and her scientific manicuring.

The texture, weight, and flexibility of the nail is determined as the cells are formed in the matrix. They depend on moisture and oil from the nail bed for their survival. Nature produces a selvage on each side of the nail. If the selvage is cut or damaged the nail will spread and fan out.

Reno taught me how to hold the emery board correctly, and to choose one that does not shed its granules as the nail is filed. I hold the file vertically against the center edge of the nail and I do not let it lose contact with the nail, as I gently move the file back and forth. This keeps the layers of the nail even and does stop the peeling.

I use only pure soap in water to soften the cuticle. I dry my fingers with a soft, smooth, thin cloth towel or a paper one. I use a mild cuticle solvent.

I hold and use the cuticle loosener with the same pressure and circular motion as if I were writing with a pen. I do not deviate because too much pressure and jabbing at the cuticle will cause horizontal ridges in the nail surface. I do not let the cuticle loosener lose contact with the nail as I work up along the sides and across the moon area. I reverse the circular motion as I work up the other side. I wash away the debris and dry. Then I wrap a wisp of pure cotton over the end of a very thin orangewood stick, dampen it, and then I circle the nail under the cuticle to wipe away the film.

I use only fine, thin cuticle scissors to remove the frayed skin and broken cuticle. It is also important to clean under the nail correctly. Now I use a tool with a thin round point. I start at the corners of the nail and draw the tool to the center, then across the center to finish. If I start at the center and force the debris to the side, it will discourage the selvage from tightening the nail to the nail bed.

The proper method of buffing my nails helps harden the nail surface and stimulates the flow of moisture and oil to the nail bed. With or without a buffing compound, I place the buffer on the center of my nail and I do not let it lose contact with my nail as I gently move the buffer back and forth across my nails.

What Reno explained to me did work.

MENDING A BROKEN NAIL

Reno and I use very fine, thin coffee filter papers or the paper from an unused tea bag. These papers are very strong and porous. They are softer and more pliable then most others. Always tear the paper; this pulls the fibers, thinning and fraying out the edges. For safety and durability, use only a cement recommended by your chemist.

For a break that has traveled halfway across the nail, tear a strip of paper the width of the break and about an inch long. Apply a large drop of cement, then turn it over on your finger to force the cement up through the pores of the paper (this seals out any air bubbles). Add more cement and lace it through the break, smooth one end over half the body of the nail, fold the other end up over the nail and smooth it out. Use the orange-wood stick and more cement to work the fringe of the paper down along the side of the nail and under the tip. Tear another tiny piece of paper, add cement, place half of the length on the nail, tuck the other end over the side at the breaking point, and work it under the nail. Be sure it is smooth and *is not cemented to the skin.*

TO REPLACE A NAIL

Clean it with pure acetone, and soften it in warm water. Place the nail on a firm surface, use the cuticle loosener to scrape the inside of the nail free from ridges, film, or high spots. Apply cement, place it on the nail just above the free edge. Hold it firm to set the cement. If the demarcation seems thick, use the emery board to file it smooth. Use the tiny paper method, where the nail is attached, on each side.

If a nail, even your own, is rejected (doesn't take), use a strip of paper with the cement, and place it across the free edge of the nail. Again clean the piece of nail with acetone. Then apply more cement, and press it down over the paper on your nail. Use the small papers on each side of the nail to finish.

Do not try to use polish remover. If you do, the cement will become gummy and it will neutralize the holding durability of the cement.

Even in the most skillful hands, Reno does not recommend the fast-setting glue, because it can dry too quickly and cause problems.

Hair Care

SHAMPOO AND RINSE TECHNIQUES

I've been using Reno's suggested shampoo and rinse method successfully. So we are passing it on to you.

I use a hard rubber comb, and a natural boar-bristle brush because they are more gentle to my hair.

Before washing your hair comb out all the tangles. Then brush up away from the hairline toward the crown of the head.

Thoroughly wet your hair with a spray or under the faucet in the kitchen sink. Apply a good shampoo that is designed for the type of hair that you have: oily, dry, or normal. With your fingers, start below the hairline over the temples. Work in a gentle but firm circular motion all the way up to the crown. Then rest your thumbs on the temples. Work up from the hairline across the forehead to the crown. Then, with the thumbs, work in a circular motion up over the top of the ears to the crown. Continue using the thumbs and work down the hairline on the neck area, giving a little more pressure over the vertebrae at the base of the skull as you work back to the crown. Always work from the hairline up to the crown. Use of the circular motion stimulates the flow of blood and relaxes the nerve endings at the base of the skull. Rinse out all the suds with water as hot as you would be comfortable. Repeat with fresh shampoo and the same pattern of motion. Rinse long enough to be sure all traces of shampoo have left the hair shafts. The hair should squeak from the hairline to the tip ends, if it is clean.

Things you should not do: Never, never rub hard over the top or crown of the head; the pressure forces the blood away from the nerve endings and can create a mild headache. Regardless how soiled, oily, or dirty your hair becomes, hard rubbing will not help clean the strands of hair.

Towel-drying the hair is just as important as the circular motion used in cleaning the hair. Place a towel over your head and let it absorb the excess water; then place another dry towel over your head and work from the hairline up until the hair is only damp; then use rollers or blow-dry.

This regime for shampoo gives the hair more luster and bounce, and affords a scalp massage at the same time.

There are many special rinses on the market. However, there are also several home-style rinses. (1) Apple cider vinegar. Dilute one-half cup to a pint of water. Rinse as needed; if the hair is clean it will not hold the odor. Continue rinsing until the odor has vanished. (2) Lemon rinse is a wonderful, refreshing rinse, as well. Be sure all the pulp and seeds are strained out before you add it to warm water. Pour a tiny amount on the hair, and work it through the strands of the hair until you have used a pint or more. Then rinse with water until the fragrance is no longer detectable. Leaving the lemon juice or its particles on the hair shaft will, in time, cause blisters, destroying the shinglelike layers of the hair shaft, ultimately breaking apart the strands. The acid in the lemon forces the shingles open, and, like your fingernails, the layers will not grow back together. (3) Chamomile tea. Do not use on white, gray, or platinum-colored hair. There are many fine types of rinses for these colors—be they natural or bottled in origin. On other chemically colored or natural hair color, chamomile works like a charm. It helps to seal and tighten the hair shaft following damage that has made the hair lifeless, dull, or mousy colored. To brew a very strong tea, use one cup of water and add a good tablespoon of dried chamomile. Let it remain at a gentle boil for one full minute; then cover the pot with a tight-fitting lid and let it stand and steep while you shampoo and towel-dry your hair. It should have cooled enough by then to use with a small pad of real cotton (cotton holds the moisture better than synthetic). Start at the scalp and work down the strands of the hair until you have used about half of your cupful. Now, either let your hair dry naturally (if you have time), otherwise blow the hair dry, then wet the hair again with the remaining half. Set the hair in rollers or blow-dry for an unset look. Note: Chamomile tea does not "live" long, three days maximum under refrigeration, so make only what is needed for one treatment. For very short hair perhaps one-half cup would be an adequate volume.

HINTS FOR HAIR CARE AND GROOMING

Cherie, my friend and hair dresser on "Dynasty" has been an expert in her field for more than twenty years. Having worked in the film industry as a hair dresser for Ann-Margret, Lana Turner, Angie Dickinson, Liza Minnelli, and many, many others, she has accumulated valuable information and tips for hair grooming and care. I was delighted when Cherie agreed to share these simple but useful hints with you.

An irritating problem that most of us have with our hair is split ends. An easy way to eliminate them is to braid your hair, in one, two, or more simple three-strand braids. Once you have braided your hair, using only your hand, gently brush upward on the braided hair. The object is to lift the broken hairs up and slightly free of the rest of the braided hair. Repeat the motion over the braid until you can see the broken hairs clearly. Then take your scissors and carefully begin trimming the clearly visible split ends protruding from the braids. *Do not,* of course, trim the bottom of the braid itself.

Trim your split ends and the length of your hair each month. An easy way to remember to actually do it is by *each new moon.* Our hair grows approximately a half inch each month (a little more in warmer weather, such as summertime), and it is good for the hair to keep it trimmed regularly. It will grow faster and look healthier.

Once or even twice a month it's a good idea to give your hair a special conditioning treatment, especially if your hair is subjected to blow-drying, hot curlers, permanents, lightening, or streaking.

Mayonnaise, vegetable oil, olive oil, avocados, egg yolks, or plain yogurt all make excellent conditioners. You can mix these ingredients or simply use one or two.

A Caution and a tip about conditioning: A marvelous way to straighten out a permanent is to saturate your hair with mayonnaise for about fifteen minutes or so, then comb out and shampoo. So if you wish to *keep* your permanent, don't condition with mayonnaise.

Whichever ingredient you choose to use to condition your hair, simply apply the natural, oily substance generously through your hair. Then wrap your hair and head in a plastic bag and then in a towel for some fifteen or twenty minutes. Shampoo twice, rinse with beer, then with clear water, and let dry.

Cherie feels that one of the best finishing rinses available is beer. After you have used your preferred shampoo, rinse your hair with beer, then thoroughly rinse out the beer as well.

Beer is also a terrific setting lotion for regular or hot curlers. It will add more body and curl.

If you'd like fuller-looking hair, then Cherie and I recommend twisting strands of hair before rolling them onto your regular or hot curlers.

For men and women whose hair is thinning, Cherie suggests a simple process at bedtime or in the morning. Simply gather a section of hair between your fingers, close to the scalp. Gently pull (from the base of the scalp) up, and then release. Repeat this pull and release motion several times, then take another section of hair and do the same thing until you have covered every section of your head. In essence this will increase the natural "feeding" process to the hair follicles and will eventually thicken your hair.

Diet

Before we actually begin this diet section, I suggest that you go to the kitchen and prepare yourself a light snack. Assemble something healthy, like carrot sticks and celery. It may sound silly, but I'm serious, because I've found that as you dig around in this highly sensitive area (overeating, and the probable reason for doing so), it can make you very hungry.

What is food taking the place of in your life? Most women I've known have been overweight because of emotional or psychological problems.

All of my life, I have been blessed with a wonderful metabolism. However, I have to be careful not to overeat, just like anyone else.

In the past, when faced with emotionally devastating situations, I tended to become a mere skeleton of myself; I would lose weight as opposed to gaining. Either can be equally unattractive and unhealthy.

Since I've been working on the television series "Dynasty," I've noticed that when I'm doing highly emotional scenes, I want to feed myself more than usual.

Considering the character I play on the show (a woman who's suffering a great deal of the time, who doesn't receive the love she so desperately needs), it really isn't surprising that I want to comfort myself with food.

What I find interesting about my behavior is the type of food I crave. I don't want my usual favorites, or something healthy. I need *family foods, comforting foods,* things that my mother used to give me when I was a little girl.

In so many cases, food is replacing love in our minds. When we were children and something had hurt us, we'd scream and cry for our mothers to pick us up. But more often than not, instead of a hug Mom would say, "Here, have some chocolates or sweets. Do you want some biscuits?" So we must find other ways to ease the pain. Ways that do not add to our unhappiness, the way being out of shape does. Eating, at very best, is just sublimating but not removing the emotional pain, or even improving the situation.

We cannot give food power over us! I don't, simply because I have learned to love myself far more than I ever could love food.

When something hurts me or is emotionally disturbing, I acknowledge the pain. But I never use food to soothe it. Instead, I communicate directly with my inner self, not through my mouth, not through food, but through my inner thoughts.

Often I say, Sure it hurts, it feels miserable. But I'm doing the best I can. And if I eat, the problem will still be there when I'm through. I don't have to stuff myself and end up feeling sick and fat. All eating will do is make me angry and unhappy with myself.

We must take the time to understand our eating patterns. We must try to recognize when we are using food to replace love, sex, companionship, or to combat feelings of rejection.

As children we don't understand what is happening to us. The sugar tastes good, and that's better than nothing at all. But it is not what we wanted in the first place. And all it really does is make our blood sugar go up, so we feel a little high for a few minutes.

The pattern begins.

Then as adults, when we don't get what we need emotionally (in business *or* relationships), anxiety strikes and we say, "I feel awful. I'll have something good to eat, and that'll make me feel better."

Psychologically, we want desperately to give ourselves pleasure to compensate for the pain we're going through. It's those old mental tapes replaying—tapes from our childhood. The needs of a small child, carried into adulthood. There comes a time to erase these old, unproductive tapes and make new ones.

First we must realize, recognize, that there is nothing, literally nothing, *emotionally satisfying* about food. And yet, any pleasure during a painful situation is satisfying to some degree.

Before I even begin a diet, I set certain goals for myself. And I always plan a certain special day when I will allow myself anything I want to eat. One day that I can indulge myself. It gives me something to look forward to. This removes the pressure and frees my mind to concentrate on the pleasure I derive from knowing that I'm getting in shape, and looking better every single day.

Most people have a horrible time dieting because they *lie to themselves*. They go on a diet, suffer for a little while, and then they CHEAT.

Eventually, they will resume the diet and then will cheat again.

Their bodies don't even believe them anymore. In their minds, their subconscious minds, it is known that they are lying to themselves, and that they will follow the same *old patterns*.

Once you've been lying to yourself and failing at your diets long enough, the minute you say *diet,* something inside of you replies, This is going to be another runaround. We're *really* not going to go through this. I'm not *actually* going to get thin. All I'm going to do is suffer for a while, and then I'll cheat again.

Done often enough, you create an enemy inside, making dieting impossible.

We have to learn to keep our promises to ourselves. Instead of making excuses about not having what we want, and punishing ourselves by feeling guilty every time we look in the mirror or try on clothes that are too tight, *we have to make a commitment*. Then we must keep it.

Sit down and make a binding commitment to yourself, talk to yourself: I trust myself! This time I mean it, happily and lovingly. I want to look my best, I want to go through with this diet, once and for all. And nothing, *nothing* will deter me from my goal. I will keep my word to myself.

A very good way, I've found, to begin keeping your word to yourself is to find a quiet place and be alone with your thoughts. Take a clean piece of paper and write your reasons for not being thin. Simply make yourself a special list. For example:

What is my program for failure?
Why shouldn't I be thin?
Why am I not as healthy as I should be?
Why do I believe that others can look good, but not me?
When did my weight problem start?
Do I hide behind my fat?
Why am I afraid to be thin?
Can I see myself thin?
If I can't, why not?

Am I punishing myself for something I did years ago?
Why don't I love myself enough to look my best?
Do I think I'll be losing love if I'm prettier than my friends?

Make a list, then quietly and gently answer all your questions.

Another way that works for me: Before I start dieting, I always conjure up a mental picture of exactly how I want to look. I literally visualize myself as having already accomplished my goal. It sets me in motion and gives me extra motivation to continue my work. In order to change, you must overcome the blocks.

Something else that will reinforce dieting, which has worked for me as well as for several of my friends: When pondering whether or not to place that tempting piece of food in your mouth, think about how you will feel right after eating it, or the next day. Think about how guilty you'll feel every time you've cheated on your diet. Give yourself a clear emotional picture of what you've put yourself through. Recall the days you've felt miserable about how you look and feel. Right before you are about to feed yourself, remember what it will feel like later. Run the pain and frustration of being overweight through your mind. I think that you'll find it's just not worth the distress to take in the forbidden morsel. And remember all your alternatives.

Stay conscious; don't bury yourself in emotional confusion. And remember, that chunk of chocolate doesn't have *any* secret ingredients that will cure your problem.

The actual regimens that work best for me are low-carbohydrate diets. Each person's metabolism is different so their diets should vary.

There are many diets available that will work safely and effectively. Again, for my body, low-carbohydrate diets are the best. And I make sure never to eat in excess of the carbohydrate calories my body burns in a day. Obviously, it's essential never to allow yourself to go beyond a certain weight before resuming control.

If I know that I'm going to be dieting for a prolonged period of time, I take a vitamin supplement. I am a strong believer in carefully planned vitamin programs. I know from personal experience that they can increase our potential energy. I keep a very rigorous daily schedule, and find that I feel considerably better while on my vitamin program.

Special Exercise Program with Weights

There are many good reasons for working out with weights. I started exercising with weights nearly twenty years ago. I adopted the habit because I've never wanted to spend hours exhausting myself, and wasting valuable time exercising. Using weights is the fastest most efficient way to tone and add precise definition to the body.

Recently, I've heard people say, "If a woman works out with weights she'll look like a man." Well, all I can say is, I've been using weights for close to twenty years, and do I look like a man?

One of the reasons I'm such a firm believer in weights is because I understand how to make them work for me. First of all, it takes a prolonged period of time to develop a muscle, and then additional time to maintain it. Whenever I feel that a particular muscle is becoming too large, I simply decrease, or even halt, working on it.

A well-executed weight program will not only strengthen and develop your muscles, it's also good for the circulation and the nervous system. It can improve eating and sleeping habits, as well as endurance. A well-toned muscle also uses considerably less energy when performing routine tasks.

Today, there are a multitude of wonderful spas and health clubs available where instructors can assist in arranging individual workouts. From the most exclusive clubs to the Y.W.C.A., women today have the opportunity to use weights and machines to improve the way they look and feel.

However if going to a spa or a gym isn't convenient for you, you can achieve the same results in the comfort of your own home.

Many years ago, when I was married to John Derek, I began a special weight-lifting program with his help. I needed a workout system that I could do at home, so we designed one ourselves.

For just a few dollars we made our own weights, and in place of exercise machines we came up with ways to do similar "resistance exercising" by working body against body. Once we'd perfected the idea, I began inviting my girlfriends over to work out with me every other day, for half an hour.

As you will see in the photographs, the Buddy System is a simple, quick, and fun-to-do method of exercising. Anne Randall, an actress friend of mine was one of my original exercise buddies, and is helping me demonstrate the process in the following photos.

Because the Buddy System was designed at home without any professional supervision, I decided to ask an expert in the medical field to comment on the possible problems.

Dr. Robert Rosenfeld, orthopedic surgeon and team physician for the L.A. (Oakland) Raiders football team, was kind enough to share his feelings about my program. He said that as long as you do not overdo it in the beginning by using too much weight, you should have no problem. However, if you have a history of back problems, the doctor suggests doing certain exercises to strengthen the problem areas before you begin a weight program. Doctor Rosenfeld recommended specific exercises (see pages 104–110).

The real key is to commit yourself to getting in shape and then taking your time to slowly develop your muscles. If you do, there's no way that you won't benefit from a workout program.

HOW TO MAKE YOUR OWN WEIGHTS

The weights John and I made were wonderful, because they were soft and could be strapped over the shoulders, ankles, wrists, etc. All you need is some sand (beach or cat-litter sand) or airgun pellets, some fabric or just a few old socks and some plastic bags, and some twine or string.

When using a sock (try to find one without holes in it), simply pour the sand or pellets into two plastic bags (one inside the other, double). Weigh the contents until you have the desired weight. We used 2½ or 5-pound bags. Insert the filled double-lined baggies into the sock. You will have to stretch the sock carefully over the bags. Then tie off both the socks and the

HOW TO MAKE WEIGHTS

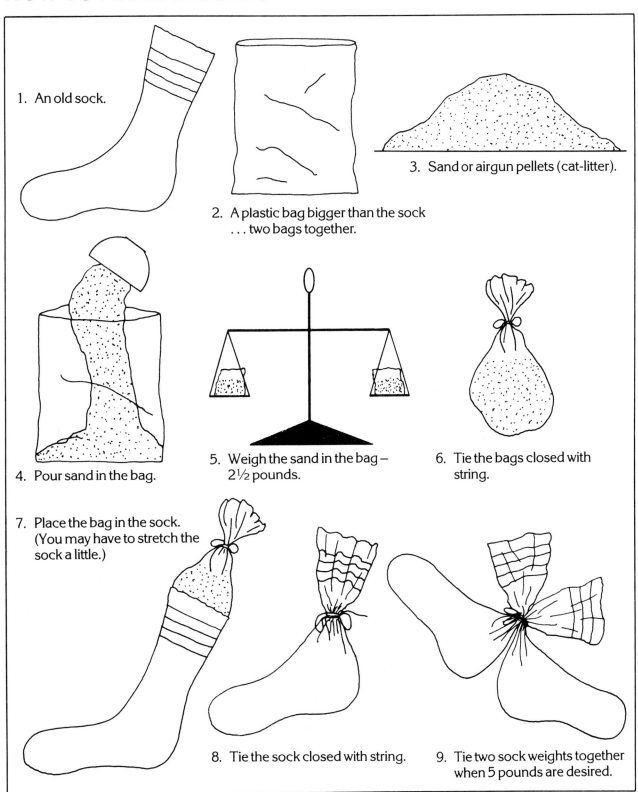

1. An old sock.

2. A plastic bag bigger than the sock ... two bags together.

3. Sand or airgun pellets (cat-litter).

4. Pour sand in the bag.

5. Weigh the sand in the bag – 2½ pounds.

6. Tie the bags closed with string.

7. Place the bag in the sock. (You may have to stretch the sock a little.)

8. Tie the sock closed with string.

9. Tie two sock weights together when 5 pounds are desired.

bags. Make a tight tie or you'll eventually have a mess on your hands. There should be enough loose material left—three or four inches beyond the tie—to allow you to tie two such sock weights together when you wish to have a 5- or 10-pound weight.

I suggest you begin by making four 2½-pound sock weights, a combined total weight of 10 pounds.

Once you have made the weights, all you really need is a buddy, a friend to work out with. Preferably someone with a sense of humor, and the desire to get in better shape with you—your best friend, or neighbor, or whomever you enjoy sitting around with. Instead of having coffee together or a card game, just plan to work out. To do something good for yourselves, and to have fun.

Allow yourself *half an hour* to work out. Begin by stretching a little to limber up. (Dr. Rosenfeld does not feel that the standard toe touch, done straight-legged, which so many of us learned back in school, is helpful.) Bend the knees slightly to ensure that you do not injure them or pull the thigh muscles. A few easy body twists, or some scissor jumps (as many professional atheletes do before competition) should be enough to loosen you up.

THE BUDDY SYSTEM EXERCISE PROGRAM

Every other day, *three times a week,* I do three sets of each exercise, with a friend. Once I have achieved my goal, I am able to lighten my exercise schedule, but I never entirely break the habit of working out. As in dieting, I visualize my goals before I begin.

When I started these exercises, I did only *two sets of each exercise;* and I strongly recommend that you also start off with only two sets. In the beginning, I found that I was extremely muscle-sore the day after a work out. You *do* want to feel some soreness (it means that you are really developing the muscles), but you don't want to be so uncomfortable that it interferes with your daily routine.

To further ensure that you *do not overdo it* the first few times, start out carefully. Do a particular exercise four or five times per set. Please don't try to see how many you can do. Believe me, the next day you'll wish you had experimented gradually. If you haven't exercised in years, it might be best if you start with only one or two of each exercise per set. As you continue to work out, you will quickly understand your body's potential. And keep increasing the weight as you develop.

Breathing properly when exercising is essential. It isn't hard to become so wrapped up in a certain exercise that you forget to take the needed breaths. No matter which exercise you are doing, you must concentrate on your breathing. It is also helpful to actually concentrate on the muscle you are working. I find that if I really concentrate on the muscle and breathing, I don't notice the pain as much.

Remember, the pain is a reminder that you are really building the muscle while burning up the fat.

My exercise routine is broken down into the following steps, because it alternates the muscles used.

1. Deep knee bends
2. Chest/pectoral muscles
3. Inner thighs/outer thighs
4. Push-ups/pectoral muscles and arms
5. Calves
6. Sit-ups/stomach
7. Back of the thighs/buttocks

1. DEEP KNEE BENDS

As you can see in the photos, I am using a 10-pound weight on each shoulder. Keeping my back as straight as possible, I lower myself slowly (never dropping or bouncing) from a standing position down until I feel the bench or chair below me. I never sit, but I do the exercise over a stationary object so that I do not drop too low. I've discovered that when I allow myself to go all the way down it puts too much pressure on my knees, which causes unnecessary irritation to the joints.

Remember to concentrate on the thighs, and breathe out through the mouth going down and in through the nose going up.

With a 10-pound weight on each shoulder and your back as straight as possible, slowly lower yourself from a standing position.

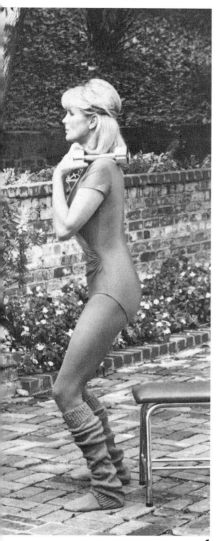

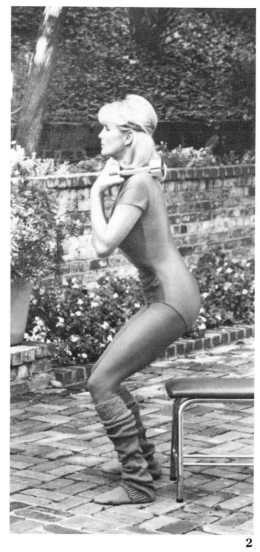

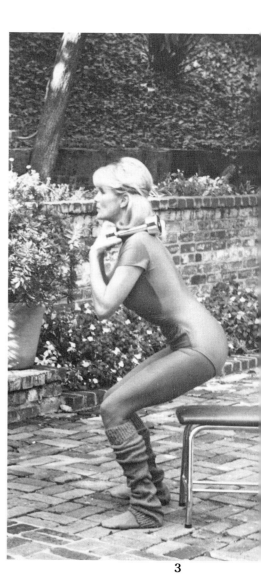

1

2

3

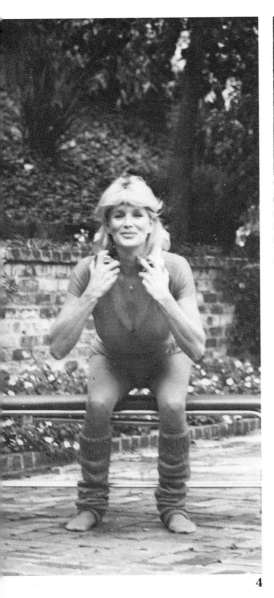 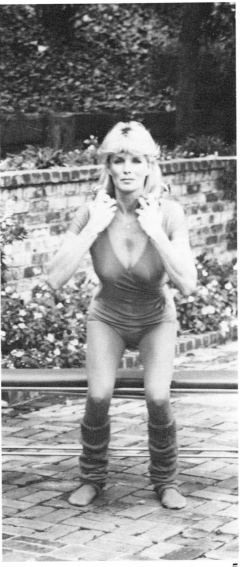 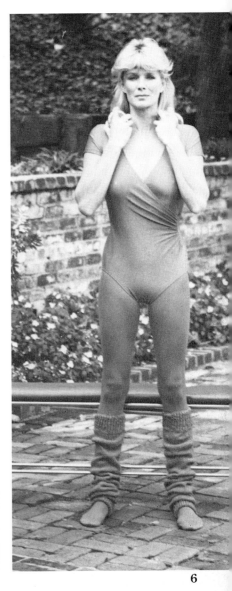

4   5   6

Exhale through your mouth as you go down, inhale through your nose as you come up.

2. CHEST: PECTORAL MUSCLES

I think this is one of the most important and beneficial exercises a woman can do for herself. Obviously, exercise cannot enlarge the breasts themselves. However, it can give the breasts a prettier shape and create the illusion of larger breasts by building up the muscle underneath, thereby making them look fuller.

If you are very small, and want to fill in the bony areas between and/or around the breast, developing the pectoral muscles will do it. Or if you are very large the exercising will strengthen the muscles that support the breasts.

In the photographs I am doing the exercise on a special bench. Before I owned a bench, however, I used to put a chair at the corner of my bed. Then while lying diagonally across the bed with my head on the chair, I did my pectoral exercises.

I do this exercise in two separate and different positions: one to build from the shoulder to the nipple and the other to fill in between the breasts.

To build muscle from shoulder to nipple, position your arms directly above your neck. With elbows slightly bent, slowly lower the weights as low to the ground as possible. (A)

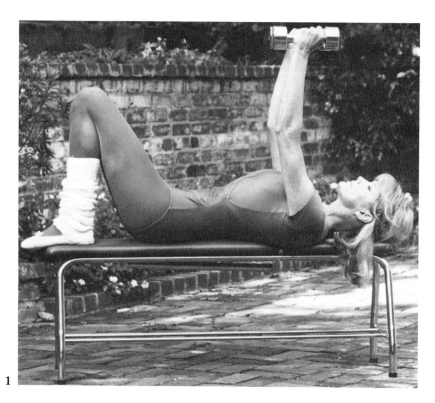

1

First position. I do the exercise with my arms placed up toward the ceiling, directly over my neck, as in photo series A. Very slowly, with my elbows slightly bent (to avoid any unnecessary strain on the joints) I lower the weights as near to the

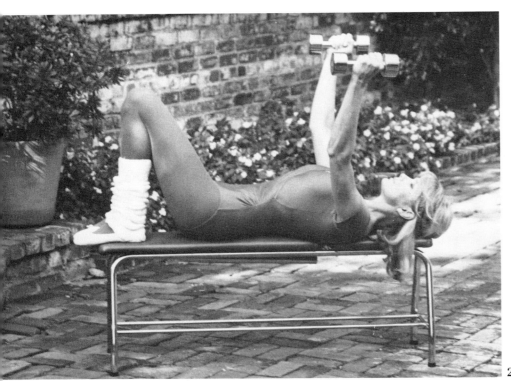

2

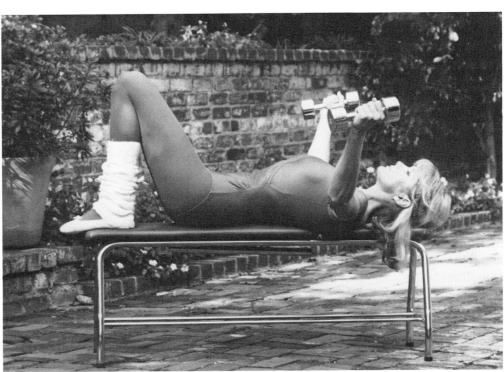

3

ground as possible, concentrating not only on developing the muscle as I work but stretching it as much as possible as I lower the weights. *Never* just drop your arms. Maintain tension and control.

Breathe in deeply through your nose, and exhale through the mouth.

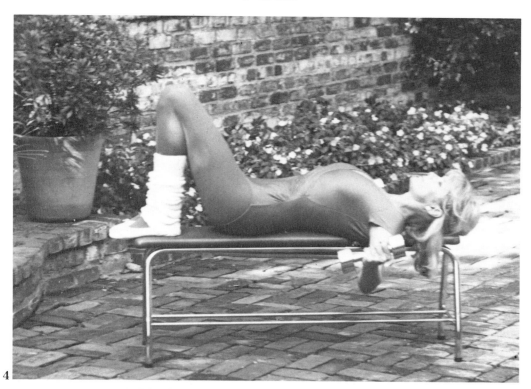

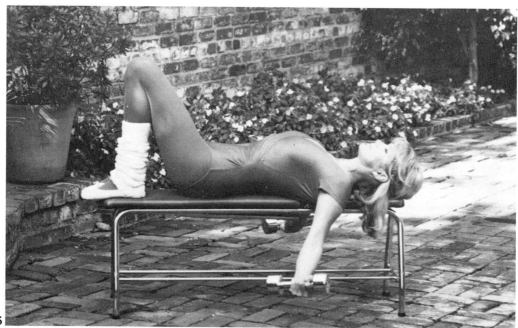

Second position. Using the same technique, I begin the weight descent from directly above my chest, as in photo series B. This will work the muscles from a different angle and will help the development lower in the muscle.

To develop muscles between the breasts, raise your arms above your chest and slowly lower them, elbows slightly bent. Concentrate on stretching and maintaining tension in your arms. (B)

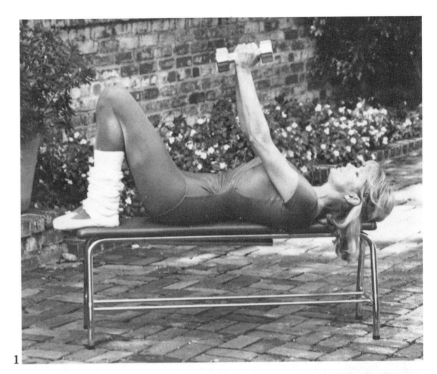

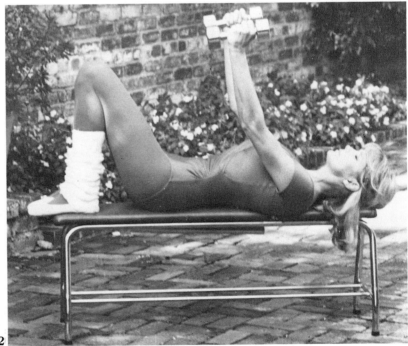

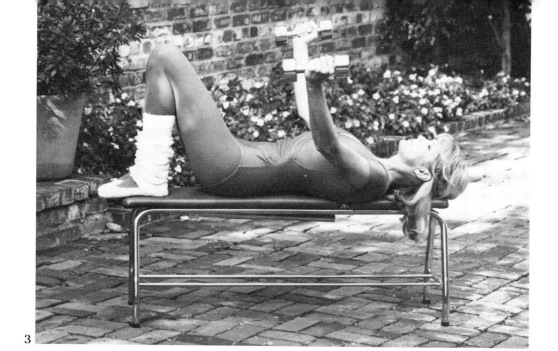

3

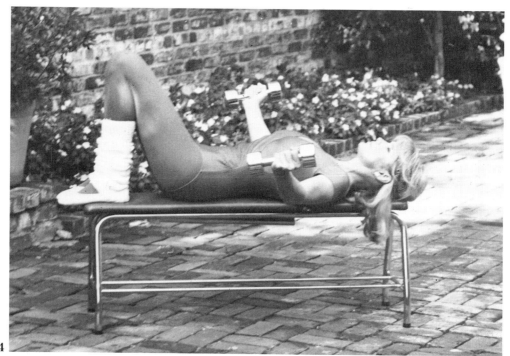

4

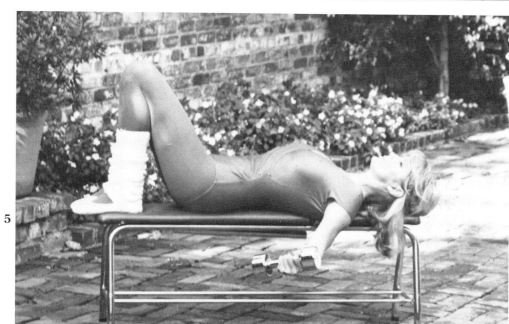

5

3. INNER THIGHS AND OUTER THIGHS

As demonstrated in the photos, the inner thigh is exercised with a friend, or buddy. Sitting on a mat or carpeted area, lean back on your arms for support and line up your knees. It is important to sit on each others feet for extra stability.

Keeping your backs as straight as possible, the person with her legs inside pushes out, using only the leg muscles. Do not raise your bodies. Concentrate on pushing out while feeling the inner thigh muscle working.

The person on the outside must allow you to open her legs. While keeping a steady pressure, she must permit you to push her legs as far open as possible. Then the one whose legs are on the outside must push your legs back together until they're closed, always maintaining the even resistance.

After you have worked out one way, reverse positions and repeat the procedure. Again, do *not* force the legs shut, or there is really no exercising taking place. *Even resistance* will develop your respective strengths and muscles.

After the initial laughter subsides and you begin the actual exercising, remember to concentrate on your breathing. If your partner allows you a steady resistance, you should be able to inhale and exhale more than once in both directions.

Leaning back on your arms for support and with a straight back, line your knees up against your partner's. Push your legs out against your partner's legs until they are open as wide as possible. Then change places and repeat.

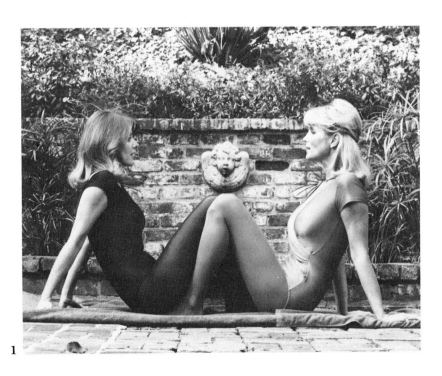

1

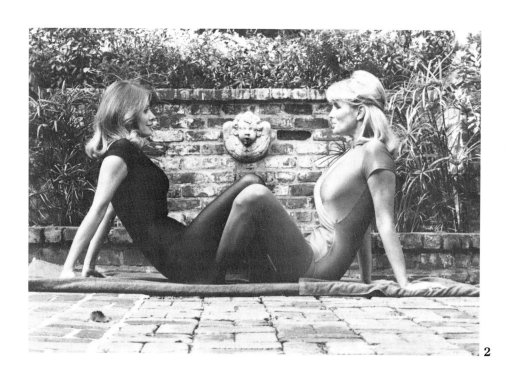

2

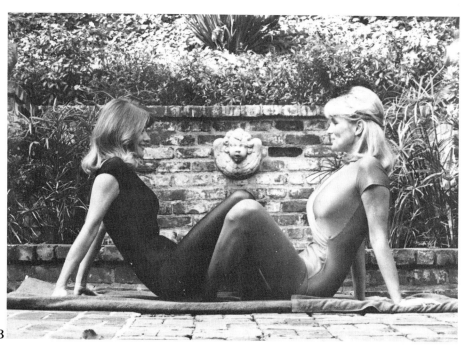

3

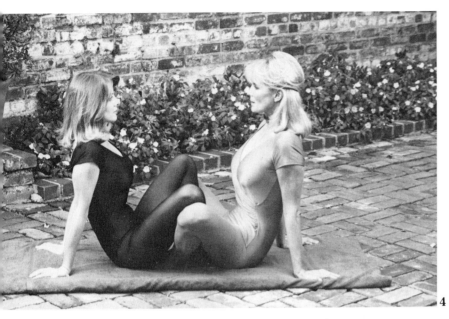

4

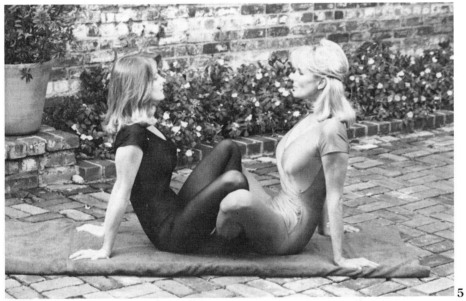

5

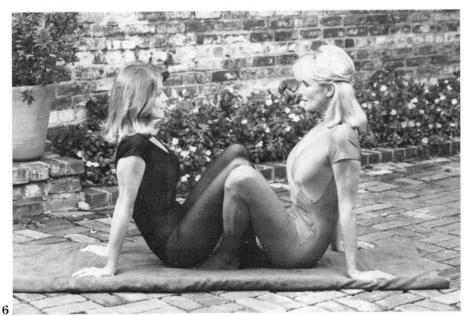

6

4. PUSH-UPS: PECTORAL MUSCLES AND ARMS

When I first began working out, I did not do my push-ups the way I do now. I did them from the knee while pushing from the arms (instead of keeping my body entirely off the ground, supported only by my toes and hands).

Dr. Rosenfeld suggests that while you are starting to develop your muscles, you can do an even gentler push-up. Simply stand 2 or 3 feet from the wall and place your palms against it; lean in and push yourself out. This will work the same muscles without the added weight.

When you do the push-up as I'm demonstrating in the

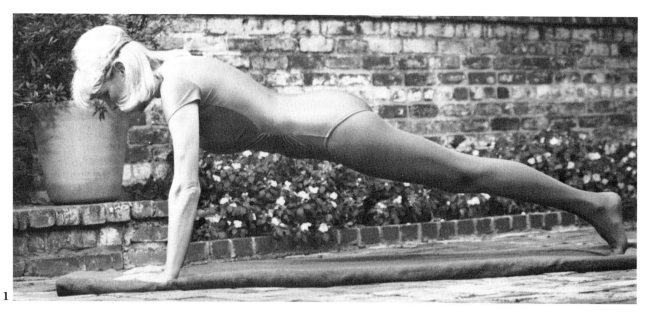

1

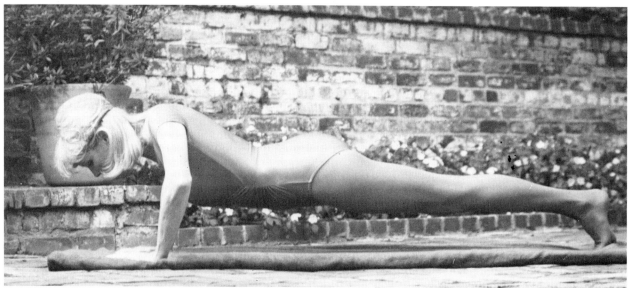

2

photographs, it is important to keep your back as straight as possible. It helps to have someone watch you to let you know when your lower back begins to curve down. Sometimes, when you are in the process of pushing with all your might, you don't realize you've let your back drop.

I find that I get the best results when I place my hands directly below my chest, with my fingers facing straight ahead of me.

I breathe deeply going up, and exhale going down. And whatever you do, don't drop down, lower yourself gently.

Keeping your back as straight as possible, place hands parallel to your chest, with fingers pointed straight ahead. Gently lower your body, inhaling as you go down and exhaling as you come up.

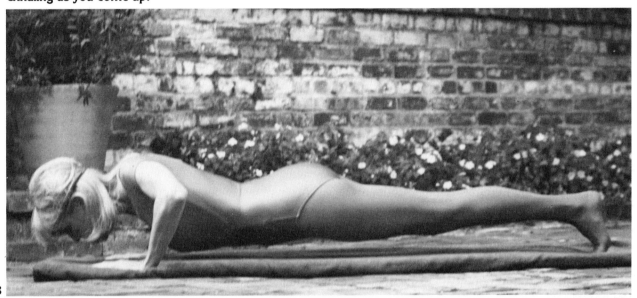

3

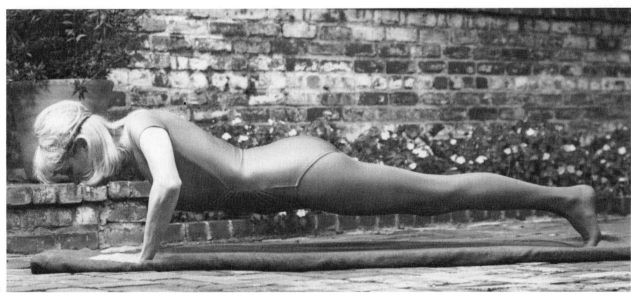

4

5. CALVES

It's amazing how quickly the calves begin to react to this exercise and definition will show. It is also amazing how fast the calf muscle starts to burn when you do the exercises.

I like to do my calf exercises with additional weight. You may find as I do that dropping 5 or 10 pounds of extra weight over your shoulders helps to hasten the developing process. It takes me a quarter of the time to really work the muscle with the weight. However, you can do the same exercise solo in the beginning. Whether you use the weight or not, it is important to do the same exercise with the feet in two different positions.

First position. With the toes pointing in toward each other, as in photo series A, lift yourself up as high on your toes as possible and then stretch down as deep as possible. You must do the calf exercise on a step or curve to give yourself the added drop needed. (Be sure you hold on to something for balance.)

Standing on a step and holding on to something for support, point toes inward (as Anne demonstrates). Raise yourself on your toes as high as possible, then stretch down as low as you can. (A)

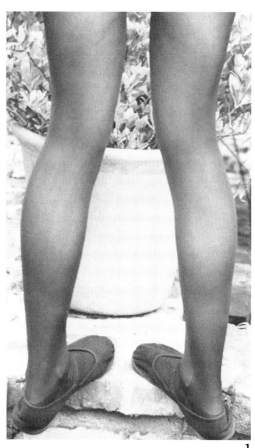

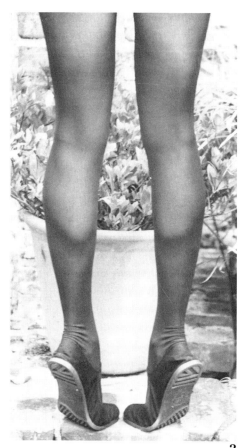

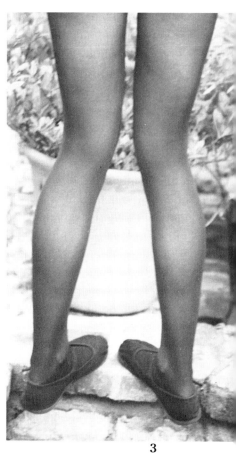

1

2

3

Second position. Do the same up-and-down motions with your toes pointing out away from each other, as shown in photo series B.

When the calves start burning, keep working as long as you can. The hot pain is proof you are building.

Point toes outward and repeat the same exercise. (B)

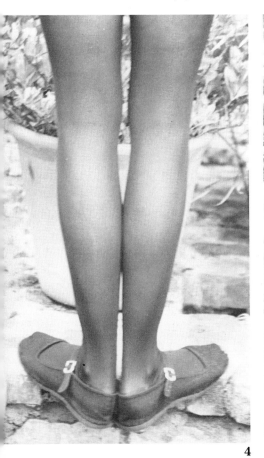

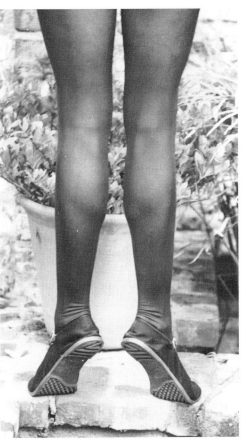

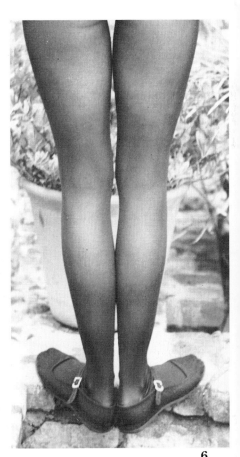

4

5

6

6. SIT-UPS

Some women are reluctant to do stomach exercises because they are afraid it will hurt their backs. In reality, one of the best things you can do for your back is to strengthen your stomach.

In order to ensure that you do not cause yourself unnecessary discomfort, I suggest that you work into this exercise very slowly. Instead of doing the push-pull rhythmic motion that I am demonstrating in photos 1–4, begin by taking the position in photo 1 and holding it. If you will simply maintain that posture for two or three minutes a set, it will build the muscles in your stomach and help to strengthen your lower back as well.

Once you have increased your strength, then work into five or ten actual push-pull movements.

Keeping your back as straight as possible, extend your arms directly in front of you, perpendicular to your chest. Pull your knees up to your chest and raise your feet, toes pointed. Slowly extend your legs and then pull back to your chest. Repeat as many times as you can.

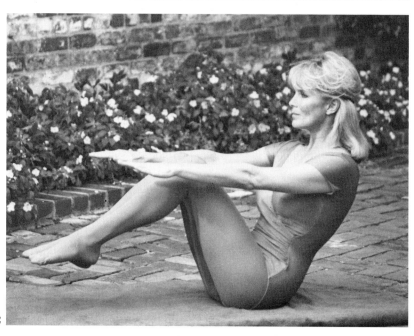

1

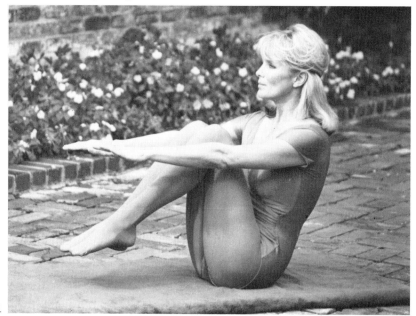

2

Sitting either on a mat or carpeted area, I hold my arms and hands extended directly in front of me, perpendicular to my chest, for balance. Keeping my back as straight as possible, I start with my knees pulled up to my chest, and my feet raised off the ground. (I keep my toes pointing out, which also helps my balance.) Then, remembering to concentrate on my stomach muscles and my breathing, I push my legs to an almost extended position (but never touching the ground), and then pull them back to my chest, push them out again, and pull them back to my chest, push them out again, and pull them back as many times as I can, which is usually somewhere between fifteen and fifty each set (depending on how often I've exercised).

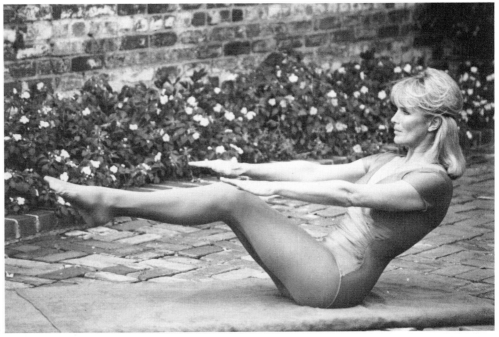

3

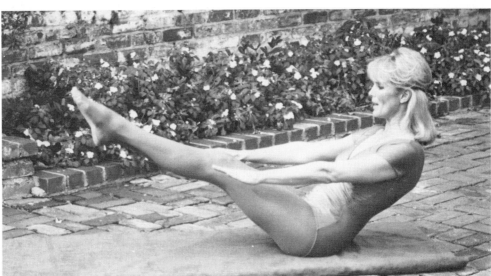

4

7. BACK OF THE THIGHS AND BUTTOCKS

This is another amusing Buddy System exercise that provokes some laughter but also produces fast and rewarding results. As you will feel when you try it, it works the muscles in the back of the thighs, and also tightens and strengthens the muscles in the buttocks.

The most important thing to remember is to keep your toes straight. If your buddy happens to push too hard and your legs can't support her, you want to be sure that your toes do not absorb the fall.

Lie flat on your stomach, your legs up and toes pointed. Your partner sits firmly on your buttocks, her knees bent, and slowly pushes down on your legs as you push up. When your legs reach the ground, return them to their original position by pushing up against your partner's resistance.

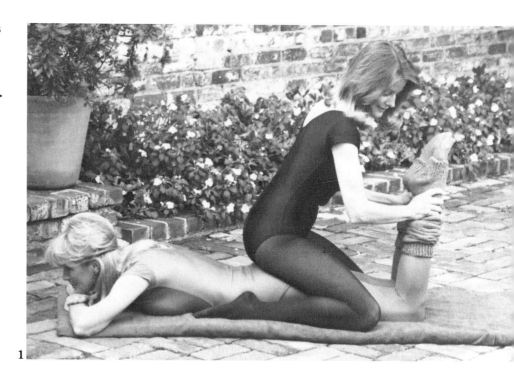

1

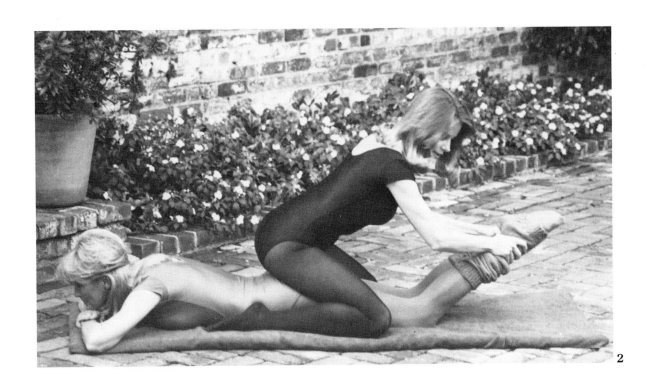

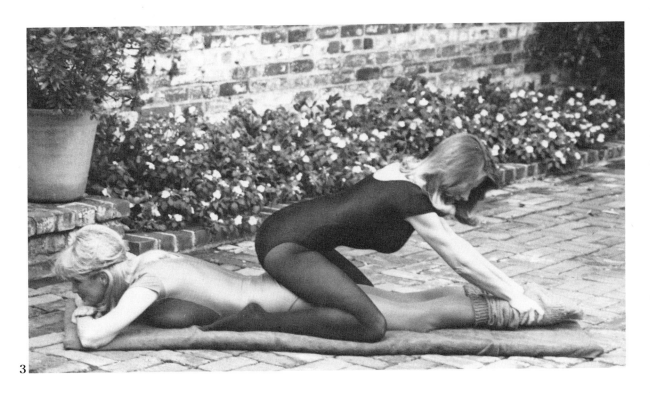

This exercise is also marvelous for the person pushing from above because it works her arms, as you can see in photos on pages 100–101. But the principle idea is to exercise the legs, so when your buddy's arms tire, he or she can also push down using only body weight and no muscle force, as demonstrated in photos below.

All you have to do is lie flat on your stomach on a comfortable surface. Your buddy then sits, straddling you, on bended knee. It is very important that your buddy sit firmly on your buttocks. It will keep you from lifting up, which is a tendency during this exercise. Keeping your legs together and toes pointing out, begin with your legs bent up and have your buddy push them slowly, but with even tension/resistance, to the ground. Do not drop your legs; fight with all your might to keep them from reaching the ground. Naturally, your buddy must allow you to descend, but not easily.

Once you are down, you must work your way back up. Again, your buddy must offer you resistance, but not too much. You must be able to bring your legs back to the original position. Remember to breathe.

When your partner gets tired, she can use her body weight instead of her arms to force your legs down.

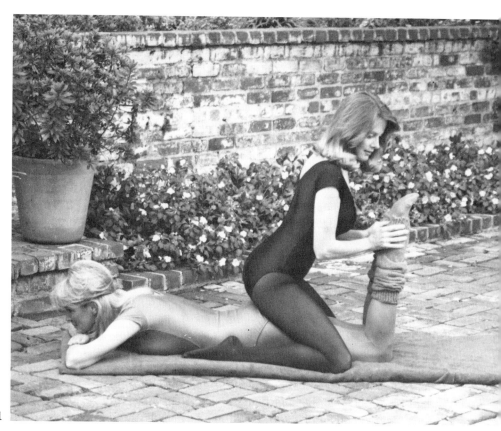

1

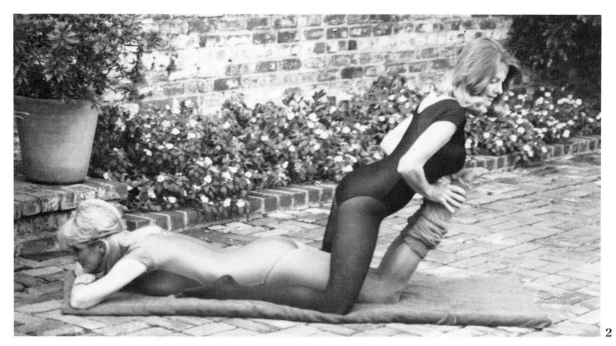

2

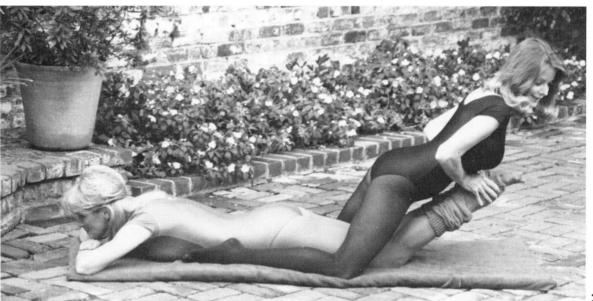

3

These are the exercises that I do. They work for me, and I highly recommend that you give them a try. When you work out with a friend, you can make it a social afternoon, laughing and talking between sets. But whether you have a friend come over, or you are able to go to a health spa with machines, or you need to work out at home alone, try at least five out of the seven exercises I do. It takes only half an hour three times a week to get into the shape that makes me feel good about myself. It all depends on what works best for you, what makes you happy.

Exercises to Strengthen Your Back

As I mentioned earlier, Dr. Robert Rosenfeld was kind enough to recommend a series of exercises that can strengthen your back and prepare you for working out with weights. You may only need to do a few of them or you may choose to do them all. That will depend on your individual condition.

Regardless of which particular exercises you elect to do, I recommend that you do two sets of each every other day, increasing the number of repetitions with each new workout.

Anne demonstrates the exercises here.

1. Lie on the floor, stomach down, with a pillow under your abdomen.

Slowly lift your left leg, straight up from the hip. Don't force your leg too high. This will cause extensive curving of the lower back.

Hold the leg up for a count of five.

Repeat the same procedure with the right leg.

Do this five to ten times each set.

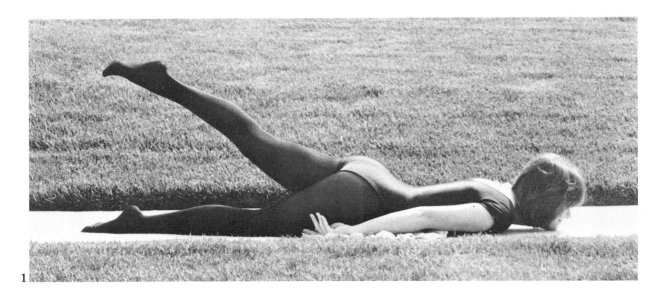

2. Lying on your stomach, again on the floor with a pillow under your abdomen, rest your arms by your sides and your forehead on the floor.

Lift your head slightly, then push forward with the top of your head. (Feel the stretch in your neck and the top of the spine.)

Hold for a count of five.

Do this five to ten times each set.

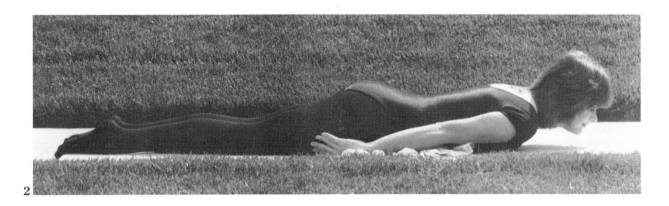

3. Lying on your stomach with a pillow under your abdomen, begin lifting your head and shoulders up and off the ground. Keep your chin pulled in, and try to bring your shoulder blades together with arms back and up.

It is also important to keep your abdominal muscles tightened at the same time to avoid swayback.

Hold for a count of five.

Repeat this procedure five to ten times each set.

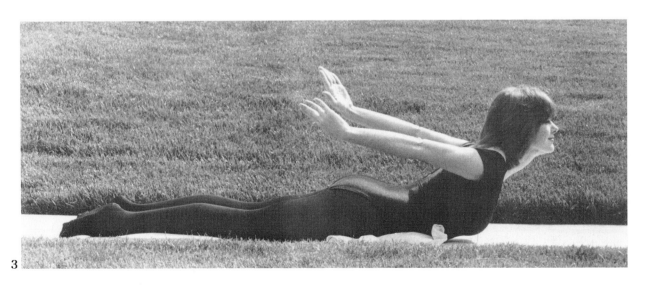

4. Lie on your back on the floor, with your head down, knees bent up, and feet flat on the floor.

Tighten the muscles in your buttocks and lift them off the ground slowly, keeping your lower back to the floor. Arms can be held up.

Hold for a count of five.

Repeat five to ten times each set.

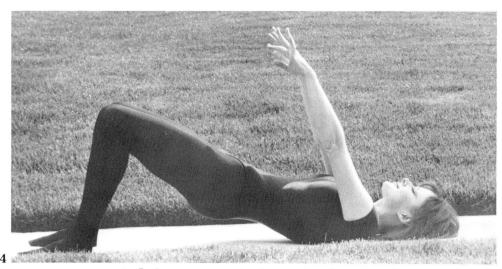

4

5. Lying on your back on the floor, bend your knees up, feet flat on the floor. From the bent-knee position, lift your legs up, keeping your lower back flat on the ground.

Return to starting position and repeat five or ten times each set.

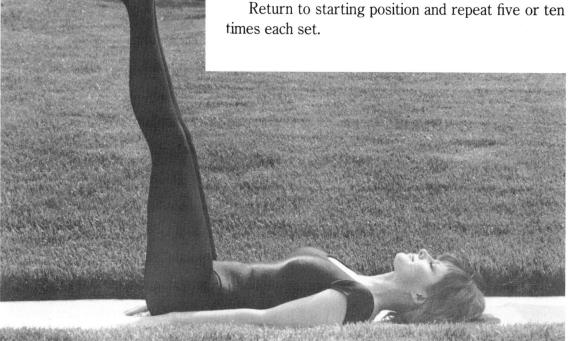

5

6. Lie on your back on the floor. You may put a pillow under your head for this exercise if you desire. Bend your knees up, keeping your feet firmly on the floor. Squeeze the buttocks tightly together. While holding the buttocks together, pull in your abdomen until you feel the curve of your lower back flattened on the ground. Don't hold your breath.

Hold position for a count of five. Repeat the procedure five to ten times.

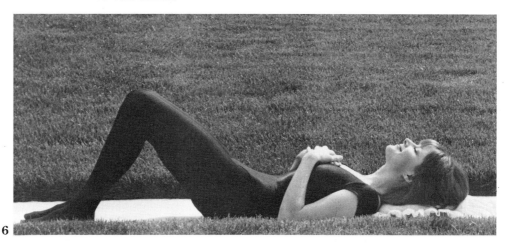

7. Begin on the floor with your knees bent up. You want your lower back flat against the ground, so squeeze your buttocks and tighten your abdomen. Then raise your right knee until it is over your chest. Cup your hands around your kneecap and slowly pull your knee toward your right armpit.

Hold for a count of five.

Relax for a moment and repeat with the *same* leg, at least three times.

Then do the same exercises with the left leg.

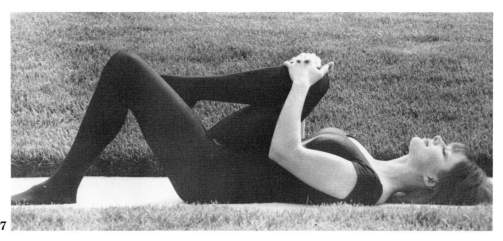

8. This exercise should be done after you have developed the strength to keep your lower back flat against the floor. Exercise 7 will quickly build your stamina, and enable you to do exercise 8, which differs only in that you keep one leg extended on the floor, rather than bent at the knee, while raising the other.

Lie on the floor with both legs out straight and down. Your lower back *must* be flat against the ground.

First bend your right knee and raise it up and over your chest. Keep the left leg straight and flat on the floor. You will stretch the hip-flexing muscle if you keep one leg straight. Hold your kneecap with your hands. Don't arch your back.

Hold for a count of five. Repeat with the same leg at least three times. Then do the same procedure with the left leg.

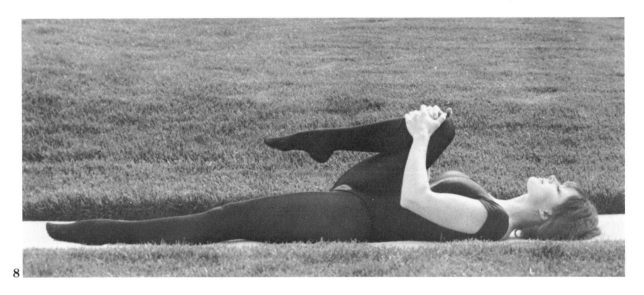

8

9. This exercise will stretch your lower back and your hamstrings (backs of the thighs).

Begin on your back, on the floor, with your knees bent up and feet flat. Squeeze your buttocks and tighten your abdomen so that the small of your back is flat on the floor.

While holding your back flat, raise both knees to your chest, cup your hands over your kneecaps, and slowly pull your knees toward your armpits.

Hold for a count of *ten*.

Return to starting position and repeat this exercise five to ten times.

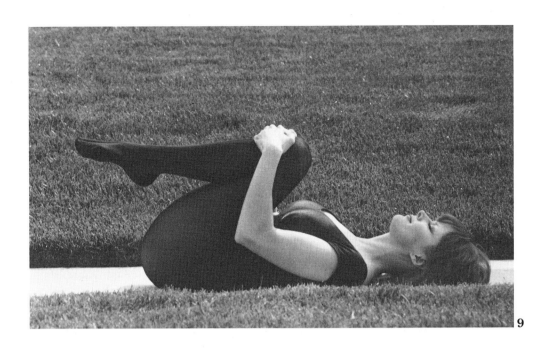

9

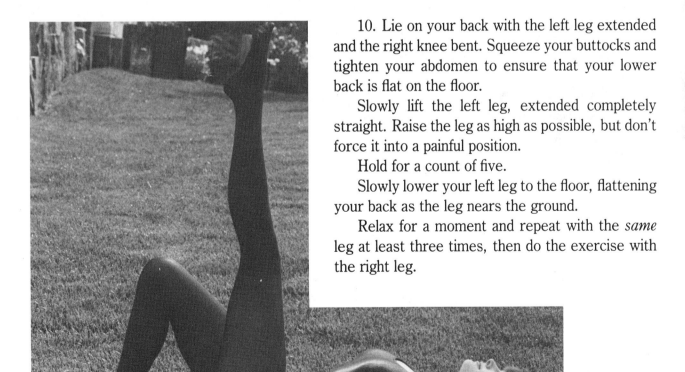

10. Lie on your back with the left leg extended and the right knee bent. Squeeze your buttocks and tighten your abdomen to ensure that your lower back is flat on the floor.

Slowly lift the left leg, extended completely straight. Raise the leg as high as possible, but don't force it into a painful position.

Hold for a count of five.

Slowly lower your left leg to the floor, flattening your back as the leg nears the ground.

Relax for a moment and repeat with the *same* leg at least three times, then do the exercise with the right leg.

10

11. It may take three or four weeks of doing exercise 10 regularly to develop enough strength and flexibility to do number 11, which is done the same way except that one leg is lying *straight* on the floor, rather than bent at the knee, while the other is being raised straight up.

Be careful that your lower back doesn't curve up (it is a tendency in this exercise). Check with your hand to be sure it isn't.

Hold for a count of five, then slowly lower the leg to the floor.

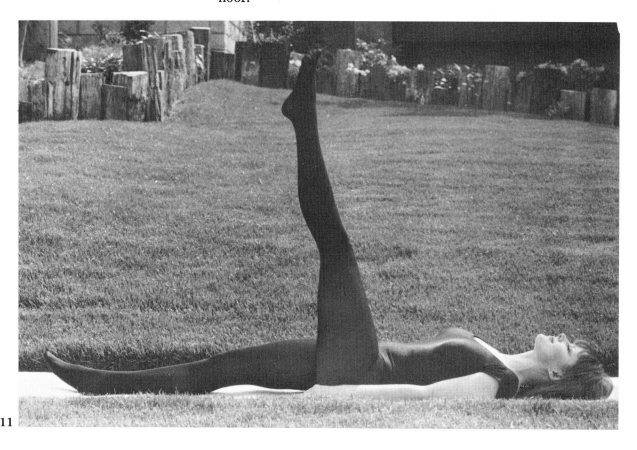

11

How to Massage Away Cellulite

There are certain areas on a woman's body that tend to produce the fat cells known as cellulite, sometimes called "starch pockets." Cellulite is most commonly found around the hips, the upper outer thighs, the inner thighs, and the buttocks. It is the rippling, somewhat dimpled fat that is so hard to lose.

Massage is the only way to remove these unwanted fat cells.

Dieting alone, even with exercise, rarely removes all the cellulite from a woman's body. But they are an essential part of the process.

About eighteen years ago, while I was working on "The Big Valley," I learned about a salon that specializes in cellulite/fat massage. I wasn't overweight, but I wanted to tone and define my body.

Since my initial visit to the salon, I have been returning on and off each year. Winnie has been very instrumental in keeping me and a great many of my friends in shape. Because of our long friendship and the fact that I know her techniques work, I have asked Winnie to explain to you how you can massage away cellulite without going to a salon, or if you're already a member of a health spa, how the masseuse can adapt her massage technique to work off the cellulite.

Winnie graciously agreed to share her priceless knowledge. However, she asked me not to mention the salon because they already have their fill of clients (most of the female celebrities in the Los Angeles area), and any "advertising" would only create havoc.

Cellulite/fat massage is not a new concept. In Europe, they have been practicing it in the finest salons for decades. Many French women help to massage off the cellulite by walking in a mild surf up to their lower backs.

The most important thing to remember is that you must exercise after the massage. You have to work the muscles to

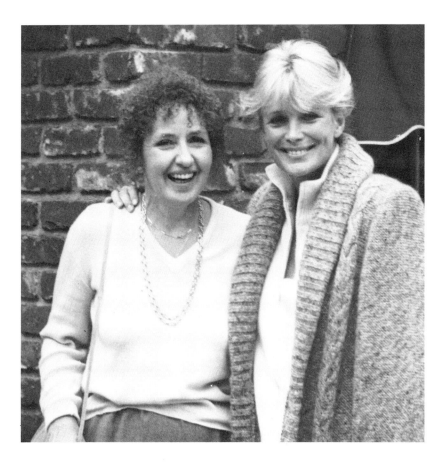

tone and tighten up the skin, or you'll become flabby. The extra
surges of blood caused by exercise will also speed up the
elimination of the fat cells.

Fat cells are not "healthy" cells; they block the normal
course of our circulation. When those areas are deeply mas-
saged *before* exercising, the cells can be broken down and
flushed out naturally.

Fat is eliminated by being metabolized and then removed via
the kidneys. Thus, it is very important to drink water when
dieting. To ensure that the fat can be quickly and easily
eliminated, Winnie suggests that you drink at least six glasses of
water each day (if not more). It is a good habit to get into in
general, but essential in dieting.

Deep cellulite massage is not painless. It is not intended to
be for our pleasure. Rather it is used for faster and more
complete results. When Winnie massages my fatty areas, it is
very painful. I compensate for the pain by reminding myself that
it is improving my appearance, and my health.

One of the first things Winnie mentioned when we began discussing cellulite massage was, "No matter how much exercising and massaging people do, they will see results only if they are seriously ready to give up the weight." She confirmed that the key to weight loss and body toning is desire. She has seen hundreds of women over the last twenty-five years come into the salon, go through the painful process, and not show any serious reduction. "They do not commit themselves," she told me. "They lose only to a certain point and then cheat on their diets. They are not emotionally equipped to be thin."

Massage, followed by exercise, will rid you of cellulite. But you must not fool yourself into thinking that you can eat more because of the massage and exercising.

When you massage, "strip away the fat layer," you are markedly increasing your circulation (especially in the area you are working on). The arteries move the blood away from the heart, and the veins bring it back. It is always better to massage toward the heart, going *up* the legs, *up* the body rather than down. Remember, help the circulation, don't go against it, whenever possible.

You can massage the cellulite while you are watching TV or reading a book. But you must remember to work out after you have broken up (stripped) the fatty cells, or you will notice that you are becoming flabbier, not thinner.

When massaging (stripping or breaking up) the fatty areas, it is important to keep your hands and skin very well lubricated. A thick body cream or even vegetable shortening works very well.

The massage is done using the same basic principle as kneading bread dough.

Begin slowly. Work over the skin lightly, gently at first. You want to encourage an extra flow of blood into the area before increasing pressure. This will help prevent any bruising of the skin.

PLACEMENT OF THE HANDS

For an effective massage placement of the hands is simple. The process will eventually strengthen your hands—an added benefit.

As shown here, take a roll of your fatty skin (stomach, thigh, knee, arm, or hip) between your thumb and your index finger. *Moving in the direction of the heart, knead the skin together, by squeezing/pushing the knuckle (joint) of your index finger over the fat, rolling it into the thumb.*

HAND MASSAGING OFF THE . . . FAT!!

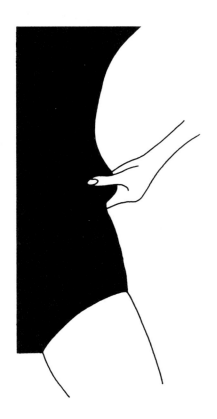

After the initial gentle start (just enough force to bring in the extra blood to the area), the massage should be vigorous enough to be irritating, even slightly painful. If it is not you are probably not applying enough force. As I said earlier, this is not a pleasure massage. But it does work, if you are willing to make a serious effort.

ALTERNATE WAYS TO MASSAGE

There are simple, effective ways to massage the fatty areas you cannot reach by hand, or when your hands are too sore to work.

Winnie has shared with us a remarkably simple and extraordinarily effective secret to massaging fatty areas with less pain and little effort. (However, you still need to work with your hands, at least on your stomach.)

You may laugh, but please laugh all the way to your kitchen, and find your *rolling pin*.

For around twenty dollars or under ten pounds, you can get half an hour's cellulite massage at a salon but you can give yourself a very powerful and productive massage using a rolling pin. I kid you not, it is absolutely amazing how well it works, and how simple it is to do.

Believe me, I had a few laughs the first time I experimented to see how it worked. It sounds absurd, but if I didn't think it was incredibly valuable, I certainly wouldn't be telling you about it.

The beauty of the system is that it doesn't take either strength or time. Simply hold the rolling-pin handles with both hands and begin rolling it over your fatty areas. Try the outer thigh as seen on page 116. Start administering about the same force you'd use if you were rolling a mound of pie dough. Increase the pressure on the upward movement (toward the heart) and lighten it going down.

I think you'll actually find it feels good. The area you're working on will quickly begin to feel hot from the surges of blood entering muscles as you increase the circulation.

As you laughingly experiment, you will see how easy it is.

For the hips and buttocks, lie on a comfortable surface and put the rolling pin under you. Using your elbows and arms for support, move your body over the rolling pin, up and down, for as long as you can.

If for some reason you prefer not to use the rolling pin for the hips and buttocks, you may do a simple floor exercise instead. (However, for the inner and outer thighs and the inner knee area, the rolling pin is probably best.)

ROLLING PIN MASSAGE

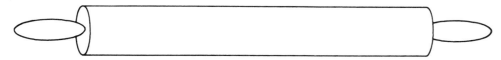

1. One standard supermarket rolling pin.

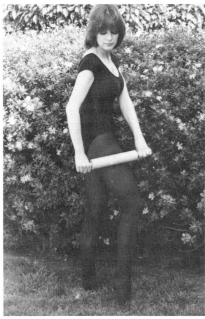

2. Use the rolling pin on your outer thighs. Up and down with even pressure.

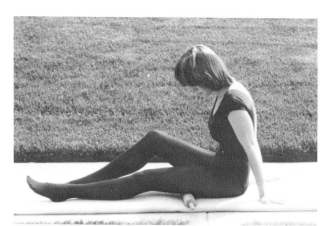

3. Use the rolling pin on the inside of your thighs too.

4. You can then sit or lie on your rolling pin and rid yourself of fat behind.

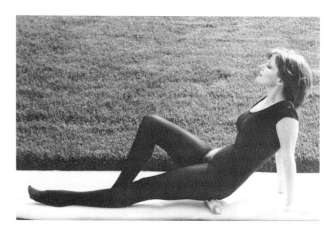

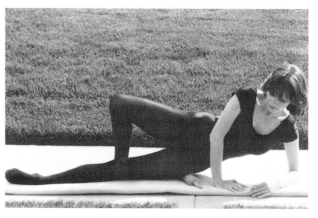

All you have to do is sit on the floor with your legs together and your knees bent up. Keep your arms extended behind you for support. Then roll your lower body from your waist, over your right thighs, to the right side, until your knee touches the carpet. Remember to keep your feet together, and try to keep your upper body as straight as possible. Then repeat the same motion and stretch back to the left side until your knee touches the carpet. Repeat the rolling motion as many times as you can. Shift your body weight so that you can actually feel the fatty areas on your hips and buttocks being compressed. Make your body weight work for you. Press your hips and buttocks against the carpet as you roll. You'll receive an extra benefit of trimming your waist if you keep your upper body straight.

Whether you can employ someone to massage your cellulite, or work it off yourself by hand, rolling pin, or floor exercise, remember: Massage when not followed by exercise will only loosen your fatty areas and make you flabbier. All the massage and exercise in the world will be useless if you are still overeating. If you really want to succeed, it will happen.

Jogging

I used to hate jogging; the mere idea of it irritated me. I'd say, "Why would I want to go and make myself miserable? My feet will burn while my head pounds and I struggle for breath."

I had painted a bleak picture of it in my mind. Then one day a couple of years ago, a friend of mine, George Santo Pietro, taught me how to jog properly. Now I love it.

The first thing I noticed after I started was how much better my legs looked. Jogging toned and tightened them almost immediately. I also felt generally healthier and my stamina had increased.

One of the problems people have with jogging in the beginning is setting too fast a pace for themselves. A hurried walk is really enough to start. Try to go about a quarter of a mile the first day, but don't overdo it, enjoy it. Find some place pretty to walk/jog and gradually build up your stamina.

If you can add a quarter of a mile to your distance each time you jog, within a few weeks you'll be able to go two miles.

It's best to jog every other day, rather than every day.

Increase your speed gradually. Speed really isn't your goal. Just find a comfortable pace that suits you. It's an individual experience; you shouldn't feel obligated to keep up with the next guy.

It's important to warm up before jogging to avoid injuries. Stretching is probably the best way to prepare yourself. The idea is to make your muscles limber and warm before starting out. But be careful not to overdo the stretching either. If you keep everything in moderation, then it will remain enjoyable.

Here are some of the stretching exercises George taught me to do before jogging.

Simply stand facing a wall, and place your hands flat against it, straight out in front of you. Then take one, two, or three steps back (whatever's comfortable for you). Keep your feet flat on the ground, and lean forward, stretching your calves. But don't force the stretch, just lean and put enough stress on the calf muscles to warm them up, gently and easily.

Another good stretching exercise is to stand up and cross your legs. Then carefully bend over and extend your hands down to your calves. If you can't reach your calves when you first try it, just get as close as you can, but don't force yourself. Eventually, you'll be able to reach all the way down to your heels.

Whatever stretching exercises you enjoy doing—the standard toe touch (which I suggest you do with your knees bent slightly to avoid injury), or the toe touch from a sitting position—try to do at least ten minutes of stretching. Even if your jog lasts only five or ten minutes, invest some time into warming up first to prevent injuries.

I think that you'll find, as I did, that you'll do better if you keep your arms and head as still as possible when you begin jogging. If your head's bobbing up and down and your arms are waving or pumping, then you're wasting energy. Try to be motionless from the waist up; only your legs should be pumping.

It's best to jog heel to toe, and always try not to pound on the ground, but land gently on your heel and lift off from your toes.

It's a good idea not to eat too soon before jogging. Actually, if you can jog three or four hours after meals or, better yet, in the morning before breakfast, you will feel great all day.

Jogging on pavement is safe only if you have the correct shoes. Several manufacturers make special waffle-style soles designed for pavement running. Without the correct shoes, jogging on pavement can be harmful. It's actually sensible to invest in special shoes, either for grass, clay, dirt, or pavement, but not imperative (except on pavement).

As long as you warm up and wear the right shoes, you should receive only positive effects. If you'll be patient and disciplined enough to spend a few weeks working yourself up to a mile, to two miles, you'll begin to understand why there are so many people jogging today.

I also find that jogging cuts my appetite while increasing my energy supply.

There are lots of good places to jog. Most high schools and colleges have tracks that are open to the public after business hours. Parks are usually ideal.

Jogging is preventive medicine, unless you go out and ignore the simple precautions.

Dressing

I first met Nolan Miller in 1964 while we were working together on "The Big Valley" television series. Today he designs the beautiful clothes I wear on "Dynasty."

Recently Nolan and I happily reminisced about our Big Valley days. I played Miss Barbara Stanwyck's daughter on the show. Nolan created all the extraordinary costumes Barbara Stanwyck (known to her friends as Missy) wore. However, my clothes were to be standard studio stock, not designer made.

At the end of our first season, Missy asked Nolan to alter some of her gowns to fit me, so I could at least have something special to wear. Finally, at the beginning of each new season, Missy would go to Nolan and ask him how many new gowns had been put in the budget for her. If it was five, Missy would tell Nolan to make her only three and design two especially for me. She rationalized her sweetness by saying, "How can I play such an elegant, wealthy lady and have my daughter in hand-me-downs?" So thanks to Missy, Nolan did design some terrific dresses for me.

Nolan and I didn't work together again until the two-hour pilot for "Dynasty." To this day requests still come in for sketches of the wedding gown Nolan created for that first show.

He has achieved great success designing for other series, movies for television, films, and award shows. But Nolan agrees that there's something very special about doing "Dynasty."

" 'Dynasty' is the first television series that has both the budget and the scripts calling for a glamorous wardrobe," Nolan explained. "For example, I designed for 'Charlie's Angels.' We had the budget and of course the beautiful women, but the scripts rarely called for expensive, elegant clothing.

"Even in the old days of Hollywood filmmaking, movies didn't demand new designs each week the way a series does."

Another challenge Nolan faces weekly is having to dress three of us, each of us with different looks, characters, and personal tastes to suit.

In dealing with my character, Krystle, Nolan has gone with a more classic look, keeping to the subtle shades and colors.

Alexis, played by Joan Collins, on the other hand, needs a

dramatic almost theatrical look. Her clothes make a bolder statement.

Pamela Sue Martin as Falon has a young, comtemporary look. Nolan designs her wardrobe in keeping with the latest high-fashion trends.

Regardless of what your taste is—tailored, or bows and ruffles—Nolan believes that if you don't feel confident in what you're wearing, don't wear it, because it won't look good on you if it makes you uncomfortable.

Here are some of the do's and don'ts and helpful hints that Nolan has shared with me over the years.

Don't buy a garment because of the "label." If it doesn't look and fit exactly the way you want it to, it can be a costly mistake. I've done it several times myself, so I know what he means. You're better off buying something from Suzy So & So that looks incredible on you than a designer original that doesn't quite work.

Also, be careful not to make the mistake of buying something just because it happened to look great in the magazine.

"Often the layouts are done very tongue-in-cheek to begin with," Nolan mentioned to me. "You have to remember that the photographer, makeup artist and the hairdresser are all trying to create a unique eye-catching effect for that picture. It's often an exaggeration of the actual look and reproducing it for real life is sometimes impossible."

If you're an experienced seamstress, or you know a qualified dressmaker, then copying the fashions you find appealing from magazines is wonderful. Nolan suggests using unbleached muslin to experiment with the design before actually cutting up expensive fabric. You may find that you want to alter the design slightly to better suit your individual look.

Try to avoid dry cleaning your clothes too often. It breaks down the fabric and shortens the life of the garment. Having your dry cleaner spot clean whenever possible will preserve your clothes.

To achieve a longer, slimmer look, wear one color, or one shade from head to toe.

When you're overweight it's a mistake to wear tightly fitting clothes because they only accentuate the weight gain. Wearing something slightly loose (not excessively baggy, either) nearly always creates the illusion of a thinner line.

Modeling my "Dynasty" costumes
as Nolan and the crew look on.

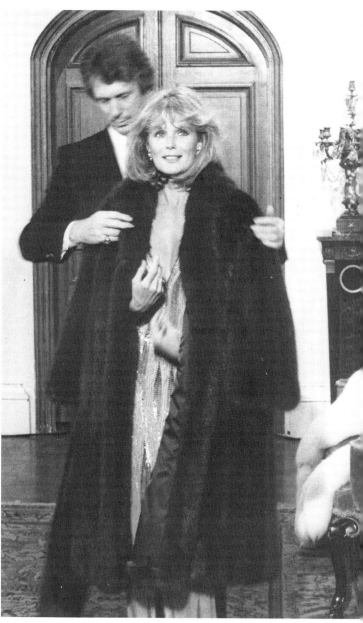

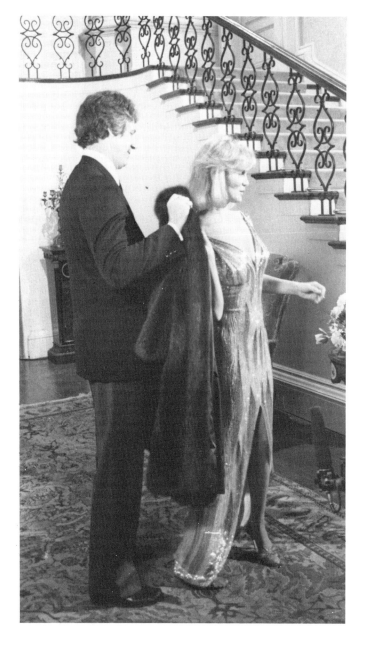

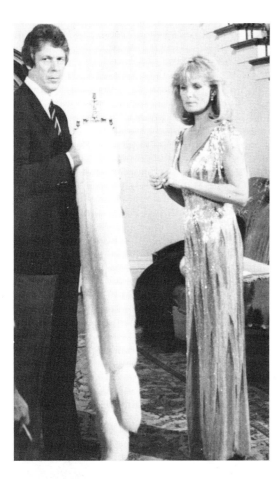

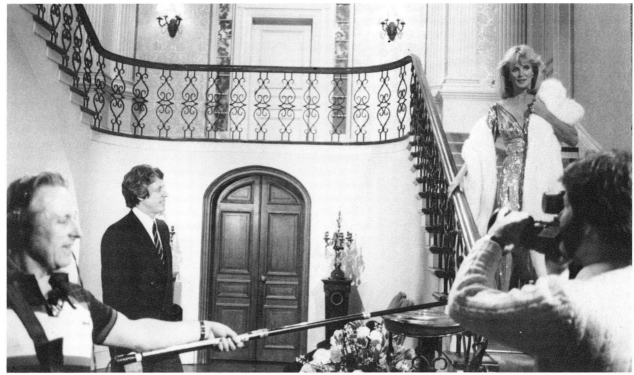

Choose the length of your skirts and dresses according to what's the most flattering look for your legs, not by the dictates of a magazine. The "in" length may be very unflattering as well as temporary. The hems of your dresses, skirts, pants and jackets should be half an inch longer in the back than the front. This will give you a more graceful line.

Take advantage of the incredible sales that come along a few times a year. It's the best time to buy the basic essentials, as well as outfits for special occasions. Even if you have to hang something special away for a few months, it's still more practical and economical than racing out at the last minute. More often than not, last-minute shopping is costly and unsatisfying.

Be aware that whatever color you're wearing will be reflected to some degree from your clothes to your face. The lighter your skin tone the more it seems to absorb the reflection.

For "Dynasty" Nolan selects jewelry from Tiffany and mixes it from time to time with paste copies of Bulgari and Cartier originals. He and I feel that today the copies are so well made that women shouldn't hesitate to include them in their wardrobe. Obviously, the paste copy has to be a fine reproduction to look authentic, but those that are well made are almost impossible to tell from the originals without a jeweler's glass. A great many wealthy women mix their fine jewelry with paste. Considering the price of insurance, it's a wise way to enhance your overall look.

To save yourself both time and money Nolan suggests investing in *good* quality taupe-colored pumps and matching bag. I know from experience that they're extremely handy because they go well with almost anything. He feels taupe is often more flattering than a bold color that draws attention to the feet.

It really all boils down to personal taste and preference. As long as you buy good-quality fabrics, take proper care of your clothes, and feel comfortable and confident in them, then it really doesn't matter what people and magazines say.

A Final Word

I hope that some of the things I've written in this book will help you to look better and to feel better about yourself. But more than anything, I hope you recognize that just where you are, just as you are is good enough. God loves you, love yourself, and let others love you . . . as you are♥